Research Notes in Plant Science

Submission of proposals for consideration

Suggestions for publication, in the form of outlines and representative samples, are invited by the Editorial Board for assessment. Intending authors should approach the main editor or another member of the Editorial Board. Alternatively, outlines may be sent directly to the publisher's offices. Refereeing is by members of the board and other authorities in the topic concerned, throughout the world.

Preparation of accepted manuscripts

On acceptance of a proposal, the publisher will supply full instructions for the preparation of manuscripts in a form suitable for direct photo-lithographic reproduction. Specially printed grid sheets are provided and a contribution is offered by the publisher towards the cost of typing. Word processor output, subject to the publisher's approval, is also acceptable.

Illustrations should be prepared by the authors, ready for direct reproduction without further improvement. The use of hand-drawn symbols should be avoided wherever possible, in order to maintain maximum clarity of the text.

The publisher will be pleased to give any guidance necessary during the preparation of a typescript, and will be happy to answer any queries.

Important note

In order to avoid later retyping, intending authors are strongly urged not to begin final preparation of a typescript before receiving the publisher's guidelines and special paper. In this way it is hoped to preserve the uniform appearance of the series.

Longman Scientific and Technical
Longman House
Burnt Mill
Harlow, Essex CM20 2JE

Hormone binding sites in plants

Michael Venis

East Malling Research Station

Longman

NEW YORK · LONDON

LONGMAN GROUP LTD
Longman House, Burnt Mill, Harlow
Essex CM20 2JE, England
Associated companies throughout the world

Published in the United States of America
by Longman Inc., New York

ISBN 0582 07800 8

Reproduced and printed by photolithography
in Great Britain by Biddles Ltd, Guildford

Contents

To Jane and to Sue

Preface

The possibility of writing a book on hormone receptors in plants was first raised (by a different publisher) at a Conference in Zurich in 1978. I declined, mainly on the grounds that there was not enough substance to merit a book. I had somewhat similar reservations when approached by Professor Malcolm Wilkins on behalf of Pitman in 1982, but after some reflection, and encouraged by the fact that the proposal was for a fairly modest-sized volume, I agreed to write something during 1984, by which time I hoped that various pieces of relevant work then being undertaken in several laboratories would have developed successfully. That the suggested title referred to 'Hormone Binding Sites' rather than to 'Hormone Receptors' was also helpful.

In the event, some of these incipient investigations have failed to mature whilst others, unanticipated at the time, have borne fruit. What I have attempted to do is review the current status of hormone binding proteins in plants, evaluate their credibility as receptors and point up likely areas of advancement. In addition, various aspects of receptor methodology have been briefly covered.

The disruption of a change in job during 1984 did not expedite production of this monograph, but the heroic efforts of Ann Morrissey and Carole Quinlan in translating my handwriting into legible copy helped to ensure that delivery was not too far behind schedule. Finally, I would like to thank those who were kind enough to discuss particular points, and also the many individuals who were generous in providing pre-publication manuscripts and information. If it seems that there is a bias towards auxins, I hope that this is no more than a fair reflection of the state of the art. Following the publishers' request for a simple index, only generic terms, e.g. 'auxin', are listed.

Michael Venis
May 1985

1 Receptor principles

1.1. INTRODUCTION

At one time a well-worn semantic debate amongst plant physiologists revolved around the expressions 'plant hormones' and 'plant growth regulators'. Devotees of the latter terminology argued that 'hormone' should be reserved for naturally-occurring compounds rather than synthetic analogues and that in plants, growth-regulating compounds were not necessarily synthesized at points removed from their sites of action, thereby distinguishing them from the concept of hormones in animals. Nevertheless, plants do contain low molecular weight substances, active at very low concentrations in regulating growth and development, that are capable of evoking responses in regions distinct from sites of synthesis. They do not seem to function as enzyme co-factors and they are active without metabolic conversion. Therefore, while recognising that there are significant conceptual differences between plant and animal hormones, the similarities are such that in this volume the terms 'hormone', 'growth substance' and 'growth regulator' will be used interchangeably. The purist distinction is difficult to sustain in any event; for example the auxin activity of synthetic phenylacetic acid was recognised long before it was found to occur naturally (Okamoto et al., 1967) as was the cytokinin activity of benzyladenosine, now known to be a natural product (Ernst et al., 1983).

Latterly the debate has evolved into a more significant one between the traditional concept of growth regulation by changing growth substance concentration and the idea, vigorously advanced by Trewavas, that tissue sensitivity to growth substances is the determining factor in plant development (Trewavas, 1981, 1982). Whilst it is perhaps unnecessarily extreme and provocative to discount altogether the role of changes in hormone concentration, the chief value of the sensitivity discussion is that it has helped to focus attention on a relatively neglected area of plant hormone research, namely that of hormone receptors. This is because changes in sensitivity, i.e. the ability of a tissue to respond to a given concentration of hormone, can be equated to some change in receptor

I

properties - their number or their hormone binding affinity. Veldstra (1956) stated the need clearly at the first international conference on plant growth substances at Wye College, with the observation that, "by dealing with one-half of the problem only (the active growth substances) we shall not be able to unravel the secret of auxin action; to achieve that aim we shall have to know more about ...... the receptor(s) in the cell". Three decades later it is a regrettable fact that our information on plant hormone receptors is still very limited compared with the animal hormone field. This cannot be attributed entirely to the relative incompetence of plant scientists, but is certainly related to the rather small number of active laboratories in this area. There are in addition, of course, particular features of plant cells - vacuolar contents and cell walls - that significantly hamper cellular and subcellular studies on labile molecules present in very small amounts.

Several animal hormone receptors, e.g. for insulin, catecholamines and steroids, have been particularly well studied, and receptor binding assays have found practical application in aiding chemotherapy and in drug design. Inevitably, concepts from animal receptor work have influenced, perhaps constrained and certainly at times misdirected plant physiological research. Most notably, elucidation of the receptor-adenyl cyclase amplification cascade for catecholamines and other hormones (Sutherland, 1972) led to numerous misguided attempts (discussed in Chapter 3) to invoke a role for 3', 5'-cyclic AMP (cAMP) as a second messenger for plant hormone action and there is still a tendency to leap on the 'messenger of the moment'. Furthermore, despite the considerable strides made in elucidating hormone action mechanisms in animals, major gaps in understanding remain. Most remarkably the central dogma of steroid hormone action, which for almost two decades has represented a classic model of hormone-receptor interaction, has now been called into question. According to the model, the steroid binds to its receptor in the cytoplasm of target cells, inducing a conformational change which is reflected in an alteration in the sedimentation coefficient from 4S to 5S. In this activated form, the steroid-receptor complex is able to move into the nucleus where it interacts with DNA and non-histone chromosomal protein, initiating transcriptional changes (O'Malley and Means, 1974). The validity of this two-step mechanism - cytoplasmic receptor binding, followed by nuclear translocation - was challenged simultaneously in 1984 by two papers using very different approaches. King and Greene (1984) used monoclonal antibodies to human oestrogen receptor and found that immunoreactivity of cells from mammalian reproductive and breast tissues was confined to the nuclei. In the accompanying paper, cytochalasin was used to induce enucleated cytoplasts from rat pituitary tumour cells in the absence of oestrogen (Welshons et al., 1984). Contrary to the prediction of the traditional model, the cytoplasts contained less than 10% of the oestrogen-binding activity of whole cells, whereas activity was enriched in the nuclear fraction. The common conclusion from these independent approaches is that oestrogen receptors are not in fact cytoplasmic and, therefore, that the translocation model is incorrect. This episode highlights the need to guard against adhering slavishly to animal hormone precedents. The precedents of greatest value are likely to be technical rather than conceptual; for example, photoactivation of α, β-unsaturated ketones, a method used to photoaffinity label ecdysterone receptors (Gronemeyer and Pongs, 1980), was the key to the first convincing demonstration of abscisic acid (ABA) receptors (Hornberg and Weiler, 1984; see Chapter 6).

1.2. STRUCTURE-ACTIVITY CONSIDERATIONS

A receptor is a specific cellular recognition site (e.g. for a hormone, drug or neurotransmitter) that binds the ligand and in consequence instructs the cell to respond in the appropriate manner to the particular chemical signal. The precision of the recognition process can probably only be accommodated in a macromolecular structure and all known hormone receptors are proteins. One of the main reasons for believing that receptors for plant hormones must exist is the recognition that for each of the six groups of plant hormones - auxins, gibberellins, cytokinins, abscisic acid, ethylene, and now brassins - there are stringent structural and stereochemical requirements for activity. This appreciation has evolved out of the physiological evaluation of large numbers of synthetic analogues, some of which have found important agricultural and horticultural application as herbicides and plant growth regulators.

Structure-activity concepts have been particularly well developed in the case of auxins, partly because this group has attracted the greatest chemical input. Figure 1.1 illustrates the structures of a few of the numerous synthetic auxin analogues, in addition to the natural compound

3

indole-3-acetic acid (IAA). The earlier attempts to define activity rules
have been well covered elsewhere (e.g. Jönssen, 1961; Audus, 1972). Implicit
in many of these was a combination of properties appropriate to interaction
with a receptor site, generally by non-covalent forces (Koepfli et al.,
1938; Veldstra, 1944 a,b; Smith et al., 1952). Nucleophilic attack (Muir et
al., 1949) and nucleophilic displacement (Hansch et al., 1951) theories,
which required covalent linkages of the carboxyl and an ortho-position on
the auxin ring with amino and sulphydryl groups respectively of a protein
were always difficult to sustain and run counter to all subsequent evidence.

Until relatively recently, the most influential of the later auxin
structure-activity proposals has been the charge separation theory of Porter
and Thimann (1959, 1965). This suggested that active auxins have a
fractional positive charge (on the indole nitrogen in the case of IAA)
located at a distance of 0.55 nm from the negatively-charged carboxyl group.
Activities of several different groups of auxin molecule, including
phenoxyacetates, benzoates and even the aliphatic dithiocarbamates
(Kerk et al., 1955) could all apparently be accommodated on a similar basis.
Farrimond et al. (1978) initially proposed a modification of this theory,
based on self-consistent field molecular orbital calculations of charge
distribution in the energetically optimum geometric conformations. They
found that if valence electrons as well as pi electrons are taken into
account, then the indole nitrogen of IAA actually bears a negative, not a
positive charge. Likewise 2,4-D (2,4-dichlorophenoxyacetic acid) was
calculated to carry a negative charge in the ring position that the Porter
and Thimann proposal required to be positive. On the other hand, both IAA
and 2,4-D, together with other active auxins such as NAA (naphthalene-1-
acetic acid), NOA (naphthoxy-2-acetic acid) and PAA (phenylacetic acid) were
found to have a positive charge on other atoms situated at a slightly
different distance (0.5 nm) from the negative carboxyl. In a subsequent
paper (Farrimond et al., 1980) it was proposed that the auxin activity
of certain nitrophenols (Harper and Wain, 1969) could be explained on a
similar basis if the isosteric nitro group is viewed as a carboxyl mimic.
However, the same report revealed anomalies when charge distributions were
calculated for some of the benzoic acid series and in a further paper more
anomalies were found when comparisons were made between active and inactive
analogues in the phenoxy- and naphthoxy-acetic acid series of auxins

4

(Farrimond et al., 1981). It was concluded that the idea of charge separation as a critical determinant of auxin activity could not be sustained, nor was there a correlation between the magnitude of a fractional positive charge and auxin activity. The effect of this series of papers has therefore been firstly to modify and subsequently to discount altogether the Porter-Thimann model. Charge separation concepts could in any event never represent more than a minimal structural requirement for activity, being unable to reconcile the contrasting auxin activities of enantiomeric pairs such as the active R (+) and inactive S (-) phenoxypropionates (Fig. 1.1).

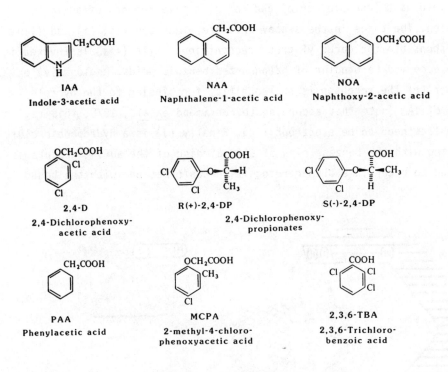

Fig. 1.1 - Some auxin structures

Veldstra (1956) concluded that, "all requirements with regard to substituents suggest they imply the absence of hindrances to the fitting of the molecule on the receptor, rather than the presence of specific binding spots". Several more recent theories subscribe to this general principle by

5

making explicit proposals for receptor configurations that would be needed to accommodate the diverse range of active auxin structures (Kaethner, 1977; Lehmann, 1978; Rakhaminova et al., 1978; Katekar, 1979). None of these proposals is without its particular difficulties, but by stressing the nature of the receptor they denote a significant shift in emphasis. The model of Lehmann (1978) is little more than a modified 3-point attachment theory (Smith et al., 1952), but the others are more ambitious. Both Kaethner (1977) and Rakhaminova et al. (1978) suggest that auxin activity depends upon a conformational change in the receptor induced by binding of the auxin molecule. The receptor representations proposed by Kaethner (1977) and by Katekar (1979) are shown in Fig. 1.2. Kaethner's receptor (Fig. 1.2a) is described as a 'canopied crib' and contains five regions of auxin interaction. The three in the canopy area are electrophilic, (i) and (ii) being responsible for carboxyl group recognition, while (iii) is invoked in order to accommodate binding of halogenated benzoic acids. Region (iv) on the 'floor' of the receptor is nucleophilic, for binding to the pyrrole nitrogen of IAA (note that according to Farrimond et al., 1978, this region would in fact need to be electrophilic). Finally (v) is a hydrophobic cleft interacting with the benzene ring of IAA. Binding of the auxin molecule is postulated to occur in a planar recognition conformation, with the bound

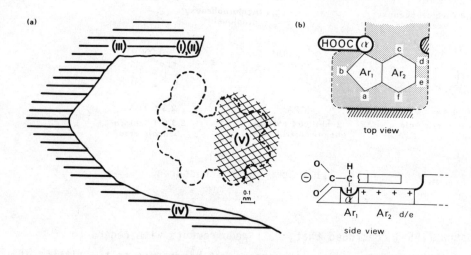

Fig. 1.2 - Models of the auxin receptor proposed by:
(a) Kaethner (1977) and (b) Katekar (1979)

molecule undergoing a simultaneous conformational change with the receptor, into a non-planar modulation conformation. Analogues unable to adopt the recognition conformation will be unable to bind and hence inactive; those that can bind but cannot adopt the modulation conformation will be either inactive or will have auxin antagonist activity. Additional postulates had to be invoked in order to account for the auxin activity of arylcarboxylic acids, since these are unable to undergo the required conformational change.

The receptor site proposed by Katekar (1979) was conceived as complementary to the IAA molecule and has IAA binding in an extended planar conformation (Fig. 1.2b). In addition to a carboxyl acceptor region and an area corresponding to the methylene carbon of IAA (α area), the receptor is considered as an electrophilic area that accepts the indole ring (Ar_1, Ar_2) and which extends beyond the boundaries of the indole ring (areas a-f). The hatched areas (Fig. 1.2b) represent regions of steric obstruction. The suggestion of an electrophilic rather than a nucleophilic ring-binding region was at odds with the charge separation theory as constituted at the time, but consistent with the subsequent findings of Farrimond et al. (1981), already discussed. Another particular feature of the model is that the electrophilic region interacts with the face of interacting molecules, rather than with the edge as in the Kaethner receptor. Based on subsequent response comparisons between pea and wheat towards 6- and 7-halogenated IAAs (Katekar and Geissler, 1983) a modification to the original composite receptor was proposed for the monocotyledon, with the addition of another region of steric obstruction in the e-f area. This, therefore, introduced the concept of subtle differences in receptor topography to account for instances of inter-species structure-activity variation.

It seems likely that a conformational change should follow from hormone-receptor binding, but this does not feature in the Katekar proposal. All the 'receptor topography' theories are based on manual manipulation of Dreiding or space-filling models. With modern computer graphics methods it should be possible to effect a more satisfactory synthesis of the composite receptor site, minimising the exceptions to current individual proposals. Ideally such a synthesis would utilise intrinsic binding activities to a known auxin receptor, rather than the physiological growth response data that have been used up till now.

For the other groups of plant hormones, structure-activity considerations have been less comprehensively developed. Nevertheless, implicit in the individual structural constraints is a requirement to satisfy demands of receptor binding and modulation, and in some cases implications for receptor conformation have been discussed.

Over seventy gibberellins are now known and Fig. 1.3 shows the structures of some that will be mentioned in this volume. Their systematic nomenclature is based on the gibberellane skeleton, to which all the natural

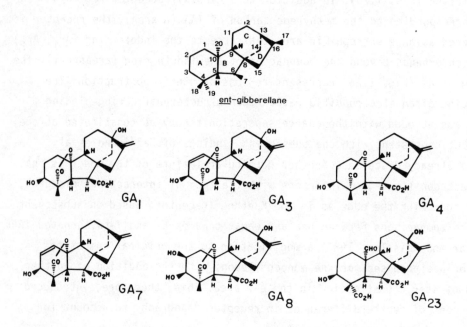

Fig. 1.3 - Structures of some gibberellins

gibberellins are enantiomeric. Routinely they are referred to by sequential A- numbers as gibberellin A_1 = GA_1, etc. The structures fall into two groups, those with the full number of diterpenoid carbon atoms (C_{20}) and those in which the angular C-20 has been lost (C_{19}). Measurement of intrinsic activity is considerably complicated by the divergent specificities of different bioassays for gibberellins (Crozier et al., 1970; Reeve and Crozier, 1974). A prime cause of this variation is probably the

8

susceptibility of the gibberellins to metabolic transformation and interconversion, particularly by hydroxylation, and the differing catalytic activities of the individual bioassay species. However, certain general structure-activity relationships can be deduced (Graebe and Ropers, 1978) and these can be summarised as follows:

1. The C_{20} gibberellins are less active than the C_{19} compounds, which are characterised by the γ lactone of ring A.

2. Within the C_{20} group, those with γ-lactone or aldehyde (e.g. GA_{23}) functions at C-20 may have reasonable activity, whereas those with methyl or carboxyl (e.g. GA_{28}) groups in this position are virtually inactive. It has been suggested (Graebe and Ropers, 1978) that this may reflect an ability of the γ-lactones or C-20 aldehydes to fit a binding area for the C_{19} lactone function.

3. A free carboxyl group at the C-6 position of the B ring is essential for high activity, perhaps suggesting interaction with a positive charge on the receptor. Methylation greatly reduces activity (Brian et al., 1967), while the activity of glucosyl esters and ethers is believed to be due to hydrolytic cleavage (Hiraga et. al., 1974).

4. 3-β hydroxylation, further hydroxylation at the 13-position and 1,2-unsaturation are all features of highly active gibberellins. Epimerization of the 3-β hydroxyl virtually eliminates activity (Brian et al., 1967). Hydroxylation at the 2-β position is a common feature of plant gibberellin metabolism (Sembdner et al., 1980), leading to inactiviation (e.g. conversion of GA_1 to GA_8). Synthetic analogues with 2-alkyl substituents to block 2-β hydroxylation have been prepared, but no clear pattern of enhanced biological activity was obtained (Hoad et al., 1982).

5. All changes in the carbon skeleton, e.g. fission of rings A and D, or aromatization of ring A destroy or greatly reduce activity (Brian et al., 1967).

Recently, speculative 'maps' of gibberellin receptors were proposed by Serebryakov et al. (1984a) based on bioassay data using a number of synthetic gibberellin analogues. The regions depicted I-IV (Fig. 1.4) represent areas of interaction involved in optimal hormone-receptor contact. An accompanying paper (Serebryakov et al., 1984b) analysed the individual contributions of 22 different substituents to the activity of 67 gibberellins and analogues in three bioassays. It was considered that the

9

additivity of the activity contributions pointed to the importance of
topological correspondence between the hormone and its recognition site.

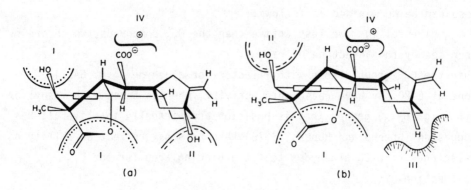

Fig. 1.4 - Hypothetical binding between (a) GA_3 and the 'dwarf pea
receptor'; (b) GA_7 and the 'cucumber receptor'.
I = obligatory binding sites. II = ancillary binding site.
III = hydrophobic interaction site. IV = site of electrostatic interaction.
(Serebryakov, 1984a)

The fungal product helminthosporol and its oxidation product
helminthosporic acid have gibberellin-like activity in some bioassays. It
has been suggested that they may represent a minimal requirement for
gibberellin activity, occupying the C/D ring region of the receptor (Briggs,
1966), but from other evidence this suggestion has been questioned (Kato et
al., 1968).

The structural similarities between gibberellins and steroids have been
frequently noted. Application of animal steroid hormones elicits various
physiological effects in plants (Geuns, 1978) and structural requirements
for corticosteroid activity have been discussed (Geuns, 1983).
Identification of steroidal hormones in various plant sources has been
claimed, though some of these claims are disputed (Van Rompuy and Zeevaart,
1979). There is, however, at least one highly potent group of steroids whose
natural occurrence in plants is now beyond question, namely brassinolide and
closely related compounds (Fig. 1.5). Brassins were originally proposed as a

new class of plant hormone in rape pollen by Mitchell et al. (1970), but it
was not until 1979, with the identification in pollen extract of a discrete

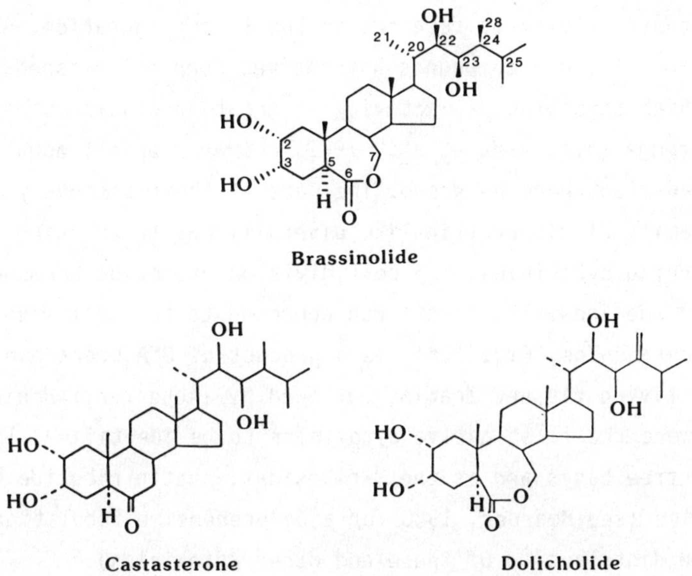

Brassinolide

Castasterone

Dolicholide

Fig. 1.5 - Brassinolide and related structures

active chemical entity, brassinolide, that this claim was convincingly
substantiated (Grove et al., 1979). Since then this steroidal lactone has
been identified from other plant sources, as have many related compounds,
bringing the brassin family total into double figures. Examples include
castasterone from chestnut insect gall (Yokota et al., 1982a), dolicholide
from hyacinth bean (Yokota et al., 1982b), brassinone (24-desmethyl-
castasterone) from several sources (Abe et al., 1983), typhasterol
(2-deoxycastasterone) from cat-tail pollen (Schneider et al., 1983), and its
3β isomer teasterone from leaves of green tea (Abe et al., 1984). Some
synthetic analogues have been prepared and structural requirements
considered (Thompson et al., 1982; Takatsuto et al., 1983), e.g. the need
for a trans A/B ring system with 5α-hydrozen, either a 6-keto or
6-keto-7-oxa function (though 6-deoxocastasterone has some activity, Yokota
et al., 1983), and 22α , 23α -dihydroxylation. Neither the 2-hydroxy group

II

(lacking in typhasterol, for example) nor the 22- and 27-methyl substituents are necessary for high activity. The nature and configuration of the 24-substituent are also not crucial (e.g. brassinone, dolicholide). Hydroxylation at the 3-position, normally α is required, but the activity of teasterone shows that activity is retained in the β- configuration. Although the precise function of these compounds has not yet been established, they have exceedingly high physiological activity in growth-promoting bioassays, in the nanomolar range (e.g. Wada et al., 1981) and are rapidly acquiring the status of a new plant hormone group. The pace of their discovery suggests that a family of gibberellin-like diversity may be emerging.

Naturally occurring cytokinins, the cell division-promoting hormones, are all N^6-substituted adenines. The first such compound to be identified, kinetin (N^6-furfuryladenine, Fig. 1.6), is a product of DNA breakdown and does not occur in living tissue. Zeatin, followed by isopentenyladenine, i^6Ade (Fig. 1.6) were the first native cytokinins to be identified. They occur both as the free bases and as the 9-ribosides; zeatin ribotide has also been identified (see Bearder, 1980 for a comprehensive tabulation of the occurrence and distribution of these and other cytokinins).

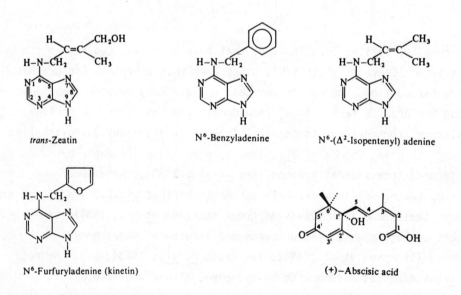

trans-Zeatin

N^6-Benzyladenine

N^6-(Δ^2-Isopentenyl) adenine

N^6-Furfuryladenine (kinetin)

(+)−Abscisic acid

Fig. 1.6 - Structures of some cytokinins and of abscisic acid

Benzyladenine (Fig. 1.6) is a synthetic cytokinin long used to support tissue culture growth, but its riboside has now been found to occur naturally in anise cell cultures (Ernst et al., 1983); the closely related o-hydroxybenzyladenosine had earlier been isolated from mature poplar leaves (Horgan et al., 1975). Cytokinins occur both naturally and in tRNA; free zeatin is almost exclusively the more active trans isomer, whereas cis-zeatin is the form found in tRNA. The location of cytokinins at the 3' end of the anticodon sequence of certain tRNA species is undoubtedly of significance in message translation (Letham, 1978), but there is compelling evidence (summarised in Kende and Gardner, 1976; Burrows, 1978) that free cytokinins are active per se and that their role in tRNA is distinct from their mode of action as cell division hormones.

The influence of structural modifications on the activity of natural and synthetic cytokinins has been reviewed by Letham (1978). Among the features important for high activity are: an intact purine ring; N^6 substitution; unsubstituted 1- and 3-positions; an optimum N^6 side chain length of five carbon atoms; unsaturation in the side chain. In addition, 4-hydroxylation of the isopentenyl side chain further enhances activity, zeatin being the most active native cytokinin. Any structure-activity model of cytokinin action must embrace the diphenylurea group. The original isolation of N,N'-diphenylurea from coconut milk (Shantz and Steward, 1955) has not been repeated from any natural source, but the cytokinin activity of this compound and of numerous phenyl- and diphenylurea analogues has been clearly demonstrated (Bruce and Zwar, 1966). Purine and urea cytokinins produce similar effects in a variety of systems, suggesting that they act at the same site. This is supported by the ability of benzylurea anti-cytokinins to antagonise the activity of both urea and purine groups (Kefford et al., 1968) and by the ability of both classes of cytokinin to alleviate the effects of pyrimidine anti-cytokinins (Skoog et al., 1973). Iwamura et al. (1980) have analysed substituent effects both in N^6- adenines and, using the bioassay data of Bruce and Zwar (1966), in phenyl- and diphenylureas. Based on steric, hydrophobic and electronic effect correlations, a tentative receptor map accommodating all three groups of compound was proposed.

Abscisic acid (ABA, Fig. 1.6) was originally isolated on the basis of its growth inhibitory properties, but it is now recognised that its most important physiological role is probably the regulation of stomatal aperture during water stress. The biological activities of numerous synthetic analogues have been reviewed by Milborrow (1974, 1978), while Bittner et al. (1977) have presented data on several aromatic ABA analogues. The structure-activity pattern is often complicated by susceptibility to metabolism during lengthy bioassays; more rapid, stomatal closure bioassays are probably a better measure of intrinsic activity than those that depend on growth inhibition. Nevertheless, the large activity changes resulting from minor structural variations argue the need for a precise molecular fit in a receptor site. Thus high activity requires a free carboxyl group, the 2-cis, 4-trans side chain configuration, an optimal length and unsaturation of the side chain, and the presence of the C-3 methyl group. Surprisingly, the non-natural (-) enantiomer of ABA has the same order of biological activity as the natural (+) isomer in many systems, though in stomatal closure bioassays (-) ABA is virtually inactive. Milborrow (1978) has proposed arrangements that permit both enantiomers to fit in the receptor site, but the divergent behaviour of (-) ABA in different assay systems suggests that there may be differences between tissues in their receptor configurations.

Although the biological activity of ethylene on plants was recognised at the turn of the century, it was more than 30 years before it was identified as a natural product in ripening fruit, and not really until the 1960s that ehtylene achieved respectability as a plant hormone. Other olefins produce ethylene-like effects, though at higher concentrations, as do some other compounds such as carbon monoxide and acetylene (Abeles, 1973). The most comprehensive comparisons of analogue activity were carried out by Burg and Burg (1967), using the pea straight growth test, from which they concluded that: i. only unsaturated aliphatic compounds are active, alkenes much more so than alkynes; ii. activity is inversely related to molecular size, presumably because alkyl substituents hinder access of the unsaturated region to the active site; iii. substituents that cause electron delocalization, e.g. halogens, reduce activity; iv. the unsaturated bond must be adjacent to a terminal carbon atom; v. the terminal carbon atom must not be positively charged. The authors showed that there is a good correlation between biological activity and the stability constants of the olefin-silver complexes and suggested a metal-containing receptor site. This idea is now generally accepted, Cu^+ being the favoured candidate (Beyer,

1976; Sisler, 1977; Thompson J.S. et al., 1983). Ag^+ is an antagonist of
ethylene action, perhaps by substituting for Cu^+ in the receptor (Beyer,
1976).

Sisler (1977) reported that a number of other compounds, e.g.
isocyanides, gave ethylene-like responses and proposed pi electron
acceptance at a metal-containing receptor and its resulting trans effect as
a basis for their action. This model therefore requires both binding and
electron withdrawal in order to generate a physiological response. Recently
Sisler and Yang (1984 a,b) have shown that 2,5-norbornadiene and other
cyclic olefins are weak competitive inhibitors of ethylene (Table 1.1). In
addition, cis-2-butene had antagonist activity, but not the trans isomer,
perhaps because of steric hindrance to double bond interaction. It was
suggested that such compounds can bind the receptor, but are not capable of
sufficient back acceptance of electrons to elicit ethylene-like activity.
Instead they occupy the site and act as competitive inhibitors.

Table 1.1 - Some olefins that are competitive inhibitors of ethylene action
            (Sisler and Yang, 1984a)

Compound	K_i * µl/l
2,5-Norbornadiene	170
Norbornene	360
1,3-Cyclohexene	488
Cyclopentene	1100
1,4-Cyclohexadiene	4650
Cyclohexene	6060
cis-2-Butene	7100

* Inhibitor concentration that doubles apparent K_m for ethylene inhibition
of pea epicotyl elongation

This brief survey illustrates the point that structure-activity findings
have specific implications for receptor topography and that this is becoming
increasingly recognised. Continuing developments in computer-assisted
molecular modelling can be expected to refine the crude pictures currently

available, but will be of greatest value when used in conjunction with information from the biological end, i.e. from studies of receptor properties and, optimistically, sequence.

1.3. HORMONE ACTION AND RECEPTOR LOCALISATION

Starting in the 1960s, abundant evidence has accumulated to show that plant hormones can elicit both quantitative and specific qualitative changes in RNA and protein synthesis. The extensive literature in this area has been comprehensively reviewed by Jacobsen and Higgins (1978) and only a few instances, supplemented by more recent information, will be noted. For example, changes in the activities of anabolic and catabolic enzymes of cell wall polysaccharide metabolism have been studied in relation to auxin-induced wall loosening during cell enlargement. Maclachlan and co-workers have conducted a detailed examination of the regulation by applied auxin of cellulase activity in the apical region of young pea epicotyls. Here, IAA induces large increases in cellulase activity and specific activity, that are blocked by inhibitors of RNA and protein synthesis (Fan and Maclachlan, 1966); polysomes from IAA-treated, but not from control tissue, were found to synthesize cellulase in vitro (Davies and Maclachlan, 1969). Later, poly (A) RNA from control and 2,4-D-treated apices was isolated and translated in a wheat germ system, and cellulase was identified in the translation products by precipitation with monospecific antibodies (Verma et al., 1975). Translatable cellulase in mRNA increased markedly after 2,4-D application, both in absolute terms and as a percentage of the total translatable mRNA population. These data are thus consistent with auxin-induced enzyme synthesis via selective gene activation and enhanced mRNA production. Another auxin-induced system, one that has no direct relevance to cell enlargement but which has been particularly well-studied in terms of auxin specificity is the N-acylaspartate synthetase of peas, which catalyzes formation of aspartate conjugates of IAA and NAA. Synthesis of these conjugates is specifically induced by active auxins (Südi, 1964) and this induction is blocked by low concentrations of inhibitors of RNA and protein synthesis (Venis, 1972). Unfortunately, failure to demonstrate cell-free activity has hindered further investigation of this intriguing system. As one further example, the well-studied process of auxin-induced ethylene production is now attributable to induction of ACC synthase, the

16

enzyme catalysing formation of 1-aminocyclopropane-1-carboxylic acid (ACC), the immediate precursor to ethylene (Yu et al., 1979).

Undoubtedly the most thoroughly investigated example of hormonal control of gene expression in plants is gibberellic acid (GA_3) regulation of enzyme synthesis during germination of cereal grains. Gibberellins secreted by the embryo diffuse to the aleurone cells where they evoke the production of α-amylase and other hydrolases that mobilize endosperm reserves. By fingerprinting and by density labelling it was first established that GA_3 induces de novo synthesis of α-amylase in aleurones, and subsequently that the time course of enzyme production in vivo is paralleled by the appearance of translatable amylase mRNA in vitro (Higgins et al., 1976; Jacobsen and Higgins, 1978). More recently, by production of α-amylase cDNA probes, it has been established that GA_3 does indeed induce synthesis of new amylase mRNA, rather than activate pre-existing but inactive message (Jacobsen et al., 1982; Muthukrishnan et al., 1983).

Modern techniques are also producing more sensitive analyses of older observations of gross auxin-induced changes in template activity and RNA synthesis. Translation of mRNA populations and high resolution separation of the polypeptide products by two-dimensional gel electrophoresis has permitted the detection of specific auxin-induced mRNA species in both soybean (Zurfluh and Guilfoyle, 1982 a,b) and pea (Theologis and Ray, 1982) as early as 15-20 minutes after auxin treatment. In soybean, IAA and 2,4-D induced the same changes in translatable mRNA species, supporting a common site of action (Zurfluh and Guilfoyle, 1982a). High concentrations of 2,4-D evoked additional mRNAs, apparently as a consequence of induced ethylene synthesis, since the same translation products appeared following treatment with the ethylene generator Ethephon (Zurfluh and Guilfoyle, 1982b). The auxin-induced changes have been further characterised using recombinant DNA methods. Both Walker and Key (1982) and Hagen et al. (1984) have prepared cDNA libraries from poly (A) RNA obtained from auxin-treated soybean hypocotyls. Independent clones containing sequences to auxin- responsive mRNAs were selected by differential hybridization and used to show that real changes in mRNA levels (rather than activation) occur in response to auxin treatment. That this constitutes a transcriptional effect was confirmed for two of the cDNA clones by hybridization analysis of RNA products synthesized in vitro by nuclei from control and 2,4-D-treated tissue (Hagen et al.,

17

1984). This report therefore provides rigorous confirmation of what has been long suspected, that auxins can produce rapid (15 minutes) and specific changes in gene transcription. Similar nuclear run-off experiments have shown that ethylene regulates gene transcription in carrot (Nichols and Laties, 1984).

The identity of the auxin-regulated gene products remains to be elucidated, but it is clear that current methodology will, increasingly, enable questions of hormonal control to be addressed with greater precision. Transcriptional changes of the type outlined require gene activation, which can be expected to be mediated by interaction of the hormone with cytoplasmic and/or nuclear receptor proteins, though release of a second messenger following interaction at the plasma membrane could also be considered.

The general gene activation hypothesis was for a while challenged, mainly for auxins, following the adoption in the late 1960s of sensitive continuous recording techniques for growth measurement, rather than the classical bioassays of several hours duration. It became evident that the lag period preceding auxin-induced growth was in the range of only 8-15 minutes and under some conditions could be much shorter. It was argued that this early growth could not be dependent on new macromolecule synthesis and indeed it seems improbable that even the rapidly responding mRNAs discussed earlier could account for functionally significant amounts of translation products within the required time. Observations of rapid hormone effects date back at least as far as Thimann and Sweeney (1937), who noted increases in protoplasmic streaming within two minutes in oat coleoptile cells exposed to IAA and the subject has been extensively documented by Evans (1974) and by Penny and Penny (1978). However, the auxin-induced rapid growth experiments had a marked impact, and allied with these observations was the renewed interest in acid-induced growth. Using peeled sections, optimum H^+-induced extension growth was observed at pH 5 (Rayle, 1973) compared with the previously determined pH 3 optimum for sections with intact cuticles. In addition, such sections were found to excrete H^+ in response to auxin treatment, acidification of the medium being detectable in 20-30 minutes (Cleland, 1973; Rayle, 1973). These observations provided support for the proton pump hypothesis of Hager et al. (1971), who had suggested, based on similarities between rapid H^+-induced and auxin-induced growth, that auxins

18

activate a plasma membrane ATPase, thereby causing an outward pumping of protons from the cytoplasm to the cell wall. The resulting acidification of the wall was considered to increase cell-wall plasticity by means that remain the subject of debate.

For a time the gene activation and rapid response viewpoints were distinctly polarised, but there has never been any reason to consider them as mutually exclusive and indeed short and longer term responses may well be causally linked (Penny and Penny, 1978). The viewpoints were in any case reconciled somewhat by reports showing that if growth rate rather than total growth is plotted against time, then two phases in the auxin-induced growth response are discernible (Fig. 1.7). For lupin sections (Penny et al., 1972)

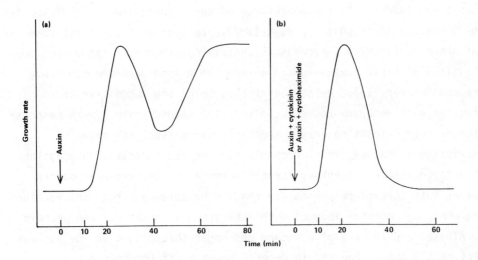

Fig. 1.7 - Effect of (a) auxin and (b) auxin + additions on growth rate of excised sections. Schematic representation of findings of Penny et al. (1972) and Vanderhoef and Stahl (1975)

the first response starts after a lag period of 14-19 min and reaches a maximum rate at 29-39 min. The growth rate then falls to a minimum after 40-63 min before rising to a second sustained maximum rate at 63-77 min. In the presence of cycloheximide, only the first auxin response is observed. The dual nature of the auxin response was re-emphasized by Vanderhoef and Stahl (1975) who showed that the second response of soybean sections could also be eliminated by the cytokinin isopentenyl adenine, while the first response was still evident (Fig. 1.7). The normal dual phase growth rate plot was interpreted in terms of two overlapping responses, commencing at 12 min and 35-45 min after auxin application. The growth rate-time curve for acidic solutions showed only a single peak, resembling the first auxin response, thereby reinforcing earlier indications that H^+-induced growth mimics only a portion of the auxin response (Rayle, 1973).

It therefore appears likely that the overall growth curve observed following auxin application is the summation of a rapid response, frequently detectable within minutes, which is mimicked by low pH, and a second response which is blocked by cycloheximide and whose timing (34-45 min after auxin treatment) is entirely compatible with a requirement for protein synthesis and indeed with the appearance of early auxin-induced mRNA species in 15-20 minutes (Theologis and Ray, 1982). The timing of the first response and of other early auxin responses (Evans, 1974), together with direct observations of rapid auxin-induced changes in plasma membrane structure (Morré and Bracker, 1976; Helgerson et al., 1976) are suggestive of an interaction with membrane-bound receptors. The second auxin growth response and longer-term effects on enzyme synthesis may reflect selective transcriptional changes, which probably require the intervention of soluble (nuclear/cytoplasmic) receptors for the hormone. Single receptor models embracing both sets of responses can readily be advanced, e.g. interaction with a membrane receptor induces both activation of an associated protein (e.g. ATPase) and release of a second messenger that passes to the nucleus and triggers genomic changes. In general however, if hormones act as allosteric effectors (Monod et al. 1963) there is no real objection to postulating hormonal receptors that are spatially and functionally distinct.

1.4. RECEPTOR CRITERIA

When studying a putative receptor system, it is necessary to evaluate the properties of the system in relation to the behaviour that might be expected of a bona fide receptor. The most commonly used criteria are:
1. Binding should be reversible, of high affinity, and of finite capacity, in order that the physiological effect can be regulated and be responsive to changes in hormone concentration.

2. The saturation range of binding should be consistent with the concentration range over which the physiological response saturates - but there can be exceptions, as discussed below.

3. Binding specificity for different hormone analogues should be approximately in accordance with the relative biological activities of the compounds - however, factors other than intrinsic activity can contribute towards net physiological activity, e.g. transport to site of action, susceptibility to metabolism, lipophilicity. A given receptor should not bind hormones of another class.

4. Binding should lead to a hormone-specific biological response. This is inevitably the most difficult criterion to establish, and is rarely addressed.

5. Binding may be confined to hormone-responsive tissues, but in plants this may be a difficult term to define - see below.

From the animal hormone literature it is known that in some cases a full biological response is obtained when only a small percentage of the receptors is occupied, i.e. there is a displacement between the response curve and the receptor saturation curve (Fig. 1.8), and criterion 2. above

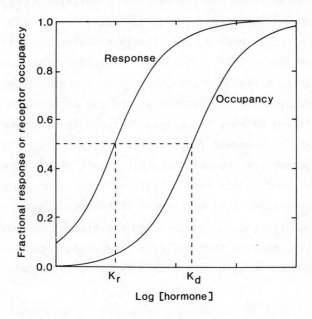

Fig. 1.8 - Displacement between response saturation and receptor saturation curves (Redrawn from Strickland and Loeb, 1981)

is not fulfilled. Proposals of varying complexity have been advanced to account for such observations, e.g. negative co-operativity, the 'spare receptor' concept (Boeynaems and Dumont, 1980), but Strickland and Loeb (1981) showed that such displacement can be expected in any system where the response is dependent upon the generation of a secondary mediator (e.g. cyclic AMP). It followed from their straightforward mathematical treatment that the hormone concentration required for half-maximal biological response (K_r, Fig. 1.8) is formally lower than that required for half maximal receptor saturation (K_d). Similar possibilities therefore need to be considered when evaluating plant hormone receptors.

Again, the normal experience with animal hormones is that receptors are confined to specific target organs, and it might be anticipated that receptors for plant hormones would be localised in hormone-responsive tissues, hence governing tissue sensitivity. While this may be so, it is not always clear what constitutes a hormone-responsive system. Simplistically, it is often equated to growth responsiveness in some form, but this neglects not only the known diversity of plant hormone effects, but also the less overt hormone-dependent biochemical changes of which we may be unaware. As an example, the auxin-induced N-acylaspartate synthetase of peas, referred to in the preceding section (Südi, 1964), is inducible not only in the growth-responsive third internode, but also in non-elongating tissue from the first internode (Südi, 1966: Fig. 1.9). The latter tissue, while not responding to auxin in terms of growth, must nevertheless clearly be regarded as auxin responsive biochemically, and can be presumed to contain auxin receptors. It may be that the tissue does not contain membrane-bound receptors essential for a growth response, or it could simply be that 'all-purpose' receptors are present, but that growth of the more mature zone is limited by other constraints such as cell wall structure. Similarly, Zurfluh and Guilfoyle (1982 a,b) have found that auxin induces comparable mRNA species in both elongating (apical) and non-elongating (basal) regions of soybean hypocotyl, showing that at least some auxin-regulated changes in gene expression are common to organs with very different growth responses.

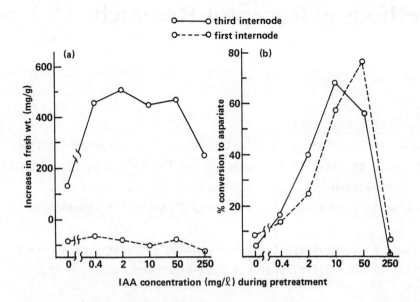

Fig. 1.9 - Comparison of (a) growth response and (b) capacity for
IAA-aspartate formation in either first internode or third internode
pea epicotyl sections following IAA pretreatment (Südi, 1966)

2 Methods in Receptor Research

2.1 TREATMENT OF BINDING DATA

The model most commonly used to describe receptor behaviour is the occupancy theory of Clark (1933), which makes the following assumptions:

1. Interaction between ligand (L) and receptor (R) is reversible. Association is a bimolecular process and dissociation is mono-molecular.

2. All receptors are equivalent and independent. Occupancy of a receptor does not alter the affinity of the ligand for the remaining free receptors.

3. The biological response is proportional to the number of occupied receptors.

This relationship is described by:

$$L + R \; \underset{k_{-1}}{\overset{k_1}{\rightleftharpoons}} \; LR \; \overset{k_r}{\longrightarrow} \; response$$

where k_1 and k_{-1} are rate constants of association and dissociation, respectively, and k_r is a proportionality constant between receptor occupancy and biological response.

Then at equilibrium, from the law of mass action:

$$K_d = - \frac{1}{K_a} = \frac{k_{-1}}{k_1} = \frac{\{L\}\{R\}}{\{LR\}}$$

where K_d and K_a are, respectively, the equilibrium dissociation and association constants. K_d is equivalent to the concentration of ligand at which half the binding sites are occupied (i.e. when $\{R\} = \{LR\}$) and, for linear coupling, is also equal to the concentration giving half-maximal response.

Since the total receptor concentration $\{R\}_t = \{R\} + \{LR\}$, then

$$\frac{\{L\}\ (\{R\}_t - \{LR\})}{\{LR\}} = K_d$$

whence $\{LR\} = \dfrac{\{R\}_t\ \{L\}}{K_d + \{L\}}$

This is formally equivalent to the Michaelis-Menton treatment in enzyme kinetics (Dixon and Webb, 1958). Converting to standard binding terminology, $\{LR\}$ = B = concentration of bound ligand; $\{R\}_t$ = n = total binding site concentration; $\{L\}$ = F = concentration of unbound (free) ligand, then:

$$B = \frac{nF}{K_d + F}$$

Commonly used linear transformations for graphic representation and derivation of binding constants are:

$\dfrac{B}{F} = \dfrac{n}{K_d} - \dfrac{B}{K_d}$ Scatchard (1949) plot (B/F vs B)

$\dfrac{1}{B} = \dfrac{K_d}{nF} + \dfrac{1}{n}$ Double reciprocal plot (1/B vs 1/F)

The binding constants K_d and n are obtained from the slopes and intercepts of the appropriate plots (Fig. 2.1). Another method, proposed by Eisenthal and Cornish-Bowden (1974) uses the direct plot of B vs F and copes better than the majority of plots with most types of error distribution (Atkins and Nimmo, 1975). In this method, straight lines are drawn for each data point (B,F) between the value of -F on the abscissa and the corresponding B value on the ordinate. When extrapolated, these lines all intersect at a point defined by ordinate n, abscissa K_d (Fig. 2.2). Other graphical methods and discussion of more complex receptor models can be found in Boeynaems and Dumont (1980).

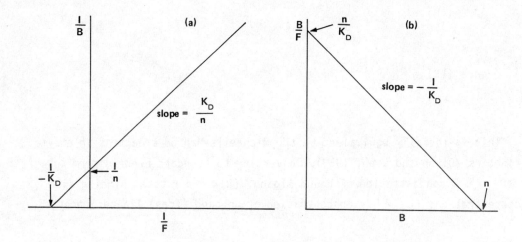

Fig. 2.1 - Linear transformations of binding data.
a. Double reciprocal plot; b. Scatchard plot

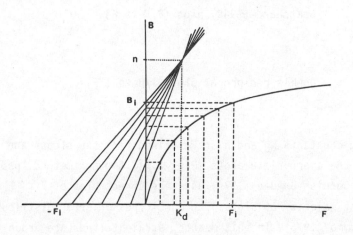

Fig. 2.2 - Derivation of binding constants by the method of
Eisenthal and Cornish-Bowden (1974)

To examine specificity, binding of several analogues to the same set of
binding sites must be compared, but it may be that only one compound is

26

available radiolabelled. In such cases the binding affinities of the
unlabelled analogues can be obtained by treatments analogous to those used
for competitive enzyme inhibition, e.g. constructing double reciprocal plots
at a range of labelled hormone concentrations in the presence and absence of
a fixed concentration (i) of unlabelled analogue, whose affinity K_i is then
given by:

$$K_i = \frac{i}{(K_p/K_d)-1} \qquad \text{(Dixon and Webb, 1958)}$$

where K_d = dissociation constant of labelled hormone in the absence of
competitor and K_i = apparent dissociation constant (i.e. -1/abscissa
intercept) in the presence of the analogue at concentration i. (See Fig. 6.9
for an example of this method). Alternatively, displacement curves are
constructed measuring binding of a fixed concentration of labelled hormone
in the presence of increasing concentrations of unlabelled analogues (e.g.
see Fig. 4.2). Frequently, the 50% displacement values (C_{50}) are equated,
incorrectly, to the dissociation constants, whereas the actual relationship
is given by:

$$K_d = C_{50}/(1 + \frac{L*}{K_d*}) \qquad \text{(Cheng and Prussoff, 1973)}$$

where L* and K_d are the concentration and dissociation constant of the
labelled hormone.

When two (or more) sets of independent binding sites with different
affinities are present, Scatchard or double reciprocal plots will be
biphasic or curvilinear. Various graphical (e.g. Feldman, 1972) or algebraic
methods (e.g. Hunston, 1975) have been described for extracting the separate
site binding constants in these situations. Increasingly, however, with the
development of widespread access to computational facilities, computer-aided
curve-fitting programmes are being used to examine goodness-of-fit of
untransformed and uncorrected data to binding models of different complexity
(e.g. Munson and Rodbard, 1980; Murphy, 1980a; Aducci et al., 1984a; Maan et
al., 1985a). These avoid the possible subjective and statistical bias
inherent in linearized transformations, though the latter may still be

27

needed to provide approximate starting parameters for the programmes. The
programmes should preferably be constrained so as to avoid arriving at
mathematically sound but biologically meaningless solutions involving
negative K_d or n values.

2.2. MEASUREMENT OF BINDING

2.2.1 General considerations

Estimation of the binding constants K_d and n involves the measurement,
under equilibrium conditions, of the amount of hormone bound to receptor (B)
and the concentration of unbound hormone (F) at a series of total hormone
concentrations. The hormone must normally be available radiolabelled,
preferably at a specific activity sufficiently great to permit binding
measurements at concentrations well below receptor saturation. The preferred
concentration range is one that will saturate from about 10 to 90% of the
receptor, corresponding to values from about 0.1-10 times the K_d or receptor
concentration, whichever is the larger - normally, though not invariably,
this is the K_d.

Either of two general strategies can be used. The first is to increase
the concentration of radioactive ligand at constant specific activity.
Frequently, a significant 'non-specific' or 'non-saturable' contribution to
the total binding is observed. In the absence of computerized data fitting
programmes, corrections for non-saturable binding are made by subtracting
values obtained in parallel assays carried out in the presence of a high
concentration (sufficient to saturate specific, high affinity sites) of the
unlabelled hormone (Fig. 2.3a). The second general method, more commonly
used because it conserves expensive or scarce radiolabel, is to use a
single, low concentration of radioactive hormone and add increasing amounts
of unlabelled hormone. Saturable binding under these conditions is denoted
by a progressive reduction in bound radioactivity, until a plateau
representing non-saturable binding may be reached at high hormone
concentrations (Fig. 2.3b).

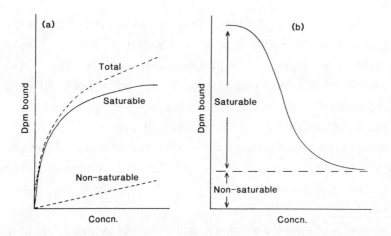

Fig. 2.3 - Binding data obtained by a. increasing the radioactive
hormone concentration in the presence (non-saturable binding) or
absence (total binding) of a fixed, high concentration of unlabelled
hormone, or b. increasing the unlabelled hormone concentration at a
constant, low concentration of radioactive hormone

2.2.2 Binding to particulate fractions

Homogenization conditions should be chosen to minimize membrane damage
and fragmentation. Pestle and mortar or fine comminution with razor blades
normally provide better results than high-shear methods involving top- or
bottom-drive homogenizers, though castellated probe homogenizers have
sometimes been used successfully. The amount of tissue used should generally
be such as to provide a final 0.5-1 g fresh weight equivalent per assay. A
typical protocol would be:

a) Homogenize tissue in 1 volume (i.e. 1 ml/g tissue) of an appropriate
    buffer. Strain through nylon mesh or cheesecloth, re-extract residue
    once or twice more in equal volumes of buffer, combine filtrates.
b) Obtain desired particulate fraction by differential centrifugation
    of filtrate (e.g. 4,000-80,000 g for a total microsomal preparation).
c) A wash step may be necessary to remove binding inhibitors, in which
    case the pellet from b) is suspended in 2-3 volumes of wash medium,
    using a Teflon-glass homogenizer, and re-centrifuged at high speed.
d) The resulting pellet is suspended once more, this time in a binding

buffer of suitable pH and ionic composition and radiolabelled hormone is added.

e) The suspension is divided into portions, to which are added small aliquots of unlabelled hormone to give a series of desired final concentrations. If organic solvent (e.g. methanol) is used, its final concentration should not exceed 1% v/v. When 'total binding' only is to be measured, then only two mixes, ± a saturating concentration of unlabelled hormone, need be used.

f) Each concentration mix is sub-divided into the desired number of replicate aliquots, generally of 1-2 ml. Binding is then determined by one of two main methods.

Centrifugation assay

This is normally the most convenient and accurate method. The aliquots from f) above are dispensed into small centrifuge tubes and the particulates are re-pelleted at high speed. The concentration of 'free' (unbound) hormone is determined by taking aliquots of the supernatants for liquid scintillation counting (LSC). If the maximum amount bound is small (<5% of that added), then a single estimation of the total concentration of labelled hormone originally present will be sufficiently accurate for most purposes. The centrifuge tubes are then drained and any adhering drops of liquid are blotted, sometimes after rinsing pellets and tubes with portions of water or buffer; the volume of pellet exposed in the surface layer is normally a sufficiently small proportion of the total that any loss of bound label during this process is inconsequential. The rinse step significantly improves reproducibility. Bound radioactivity in the pellet is then recovered for LSC by one of a variety of methods, e.g. cutting off the bottom portion of the (thin-walled) centrifuge tube containing the pellet and transferring the whole to the counting vial; resuspending the pellet in small aliquots of water; extracting the pellet in methanol/ethanol for several hours or overnight. From these determinations and the specific radioactivity, the amount of bound hormone (B) is estimated. The large majority of the papers dealing with membrane-bound sites in Chapters 4-6 use variants of this method.

Filtration assay

The labelled suspension is filtered under suction through a glass fibre or polymer filter, which is then washed with buffer to remove unbound label,

and the hormone bound to the particulate fraction retained on the filter is
determined by LSC. Both single filtration units and multiple unit manifolds
are available. This method is only suitable in cases where the dissociation
rate is sufficiently slow to permit the wash step. Without washing, blanks
and variability are normally unacceptably high. The method is particularly
useful for measuring non-equilibrium kinetics, in which case aliquots of the
suspension are normally diluted into an excess of buffer prior to rapid
filtration (e.g. Trillmich and Michalke, 1979). With polymer filters,
reduction in flow rate places a limitation on the amount of particulate
material that can be used in each assay sample.
Other methods
    Additional methods that can and have been used to measure binding to
particulate fractions are equilibrium dialysis and gel filtration. However,
as these techniques are more commonly used with soluble receptors they will
be described in the next section.

2.2.3 Soluble binding sites
    These may be either cytoplasmic receptors remaining in the high speed
supernatant after removal of particulates, or membrane-bound receptors that
have been solubilized by various means. For cytoplasmic receptors it may be
possible to arrive at a homogenization buffer composition that allows assays
to be carried out directly on the high speed supernatant. Otherwise,
dialysis or gel filtration may be necessary for exchange to a suitable
binding medium. Such a step may also be needed to remove low molecular
weight inhibitors, or these may be removable with adsorbents, e.g. charcoal.
Another effective method for buffer exchange and removal of unwanted
contaminants can be by precipitation of the macromolecular fraction with
ammonium sulphate, which provides the added opportunity of obtaining
considerable protein concentration. Concentration by this or other means
(e.g. pressure ultrafiltration) may well be needed in order to detect
binding at all. The inclusion in the homogenization medium of inhibitors of
proteolytic or other enzymes (e.g. phosphatases) can also be important.
Equilibrium dialysis
    The soluble protein fraction is placed on one side of a semi-permeable
membrane (e.g. inside a dialysis bag) and dialysed against labelled hormone.
After equilibrium is reached, determination of the radioactivity in the

31

'outside' solution yields F, the concentration of free hormone, while B is obtained from the difference in radioactivity (outside)-(inside). Equilibrium can be attained more rapidly by adding hormone to both dialysis compartments at the outset. The operation is more conveniently carried out using half-cells separated by a sheet of dialysis membrane. Various designs are available commercially, some with motors enabling the units to be rotated at variable speeds. Apart from possible complications of Donnan effects at high protein concentrations, and ligand binding to the membrane, both of which can usually be circumvented or at least allowed for, the method is reliable and unambiguous. Its main disadvantage is in measuring low levels of binding, since the B value then represents a small difference between two large numbers. With labile receptors the time needed to attain equilibrium (generally 2-5 hours) may also be a problem.

Flow dialysis

A more rapid variant of the equilibrium dialysis principle that also permits all the data points for a kinetic analysis to be obtained with the same protein sample was devised by Colowick and Womack (1969). The dialysis cell has an upper chamber containing the protein and labelled ligand, separated by a dialysis membrane from a lower chamber through which buffer is pumped at a constant rate. The rate at which radiolabel enters the lower chamber is proportional to the concentration of free ligand in the upper chamber. When enough buffer has passed to achieve a steady state, i.e. when the rates for ligand entering and leaving the lower chamber are equal, the concentration of radioactivity in the eluate provides a measure of F and, indirectly, B. Once this steady state is reached (ca. 1.5 min. in the original design), a small volume of unlabelled ligand is added and a new equilibrium (with a more rapid rate of diffusion) is reached, providing the next data point, and so on, yielding a complete kinetic analysis in 10-20 min. Subsequent improvements in design (Feldmann, 1978) allowed lower concentrations of radiolabel to be used, and have permitted the detection of higher affinity binding. The method does not appear to have been used in any plant receptor studies.

Gel filtration

Bound and free hormone can be separated by passing the hormone-protein mixture down a short gel permeation column such as Sephadex G25 (Pharmacia). Any protein-bound hormone will appear in the excluded volume, separated from the later-eluting peak of free material. Provided that the rate of dissociation is not too rapid in relation to the column run time, successive runs can be carried out at different hormone concentrations and kinetic data obtained (e.g. Sussman and Gardner, 1980). With rapidly-dissociating complexes, an equilibrium gel filtration method can be used (Hummel and Dreyer, 1962), in which the column is equilibrated and eluted with buffer containing labelled ligand at the same concentration as in the applied sample. Protein-bound ligand then appears as a peak of radioactivity above the equilibrium or 'baseline' level, followed by an equivalent 'trough' (Fig. 2.4) corresponding to removal of the ligand from the equilibrium solution within the gel as the protein passes down the column. Once suitable

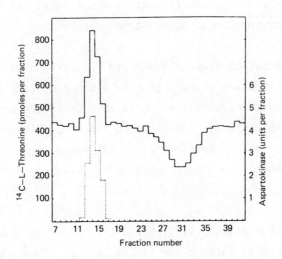

Fig. 2.4 - Equilibrium gel filtration method of
Hummel and Dreyer (1962) illustrated by
binding of threonine to aspartokinase (from Paulus, 1966)

run conditions are found, ensuring that the peak and trough are separated by a re-established baseline, then B can be measured at different equilibrium concentrations simply from the excess radioactivity in the excluded fraction, without having to determine the full elution profile (e.g. Cross et al., 1978).

Dextran-charcoal adsorption

This method has been used extensively in steroid receptor studies and has also been applied in plant receptor work (e.g. Oostrom et al., 1975). It is a non-equilibrium method and can therefore only be used in cases where dissociation of the hormone-receptor complex is slow. The principle is that in favourable cases free hormone, but not hormone-receptor complexes, bind to the charcoal. Selectivity is frequently improved by coating the charcoal with dextran, which acts as a molecular sieve and hinders macromolecule access to the charcoal. Typically, receptor and hormone are incubated at 25-37°C for 10-60 min., then chilled, and ice-cold dextran-charcoal suspension is added, the reduced temperature slowing the rate of dissociation. After further brief incubation, the charcoal with adsorbed unbound hormone is removed by centrifugation and aliquots of the supernatant are removed for determination of bound hormone by LSC.

Filter assays

These are carried out as already described for particulate fractions, except that the filter material used to retain the receptor-ligand complex is normally either nitrocellulose, which is able to adsorb proteins non-specifically, or DEAE-cellulose ion-exchange filters, which may under the right conditions selectively retain the protein-bound ligand but not unbound ligand. The latter have been used in gibberellin-binding studies (Keith et al., 1982).

Ultrafiltration

The hormone-receptor mixture is filtered through a semi-permeable ultrafiltration membrane, which prevents the passage of molecules greater than a certain size, e.g. 10,000 daltons. If filtration is not carried to completion it is possible to sample both filtrate and retained solution, giving F and (B + F) respectively. However, the method becomes very much more sensitive if carried to completion, since the radioactivity retained on the filter can then be determined, giving directly the total amount of hormone bound, after correction for the small volume of solution retained by the membrane. Moreover, the method is an equilibrium one. Usually the solution is forced through the filter under pressure, and a suitable multi-sample design was described by Paulus (1969). More recently, centrifugal ultrafiltration units have become commercially available, and these have been used to determine binding to auxin transport sites (Jacobs and Gilbert, 1983).

Sucrose gradient centrifugation

Hormone plus receptor extract is centrifuged through a suitable sucrose density gradient. Free hormone remains at the top of the gradient, while any protein-bound hormone will appear as a peak of radioactivity some way down the tube. For rapidly-dissociating complexes, equilibrium conditions can be established by incorporating labelled hormone into the density gradient, in which case binding will appear as a peak of radioactivity above the 'baseline' level.

Precipitation assays

The protein is mixed with labelled ligand and after a variable period of incubation a protein precipitant (usually ammonium sulphate, but sometimes polyethylene glycol) is added. After standing in ice, the precipitated protein is centrifuged down and the pellet (sometimes after rinsing) is then recovered for LSC. Protein-bound ligand is equated to the pellet radioactivity that is displaceable by an excess of unlabelled ligand. This method is simple and rapid, and has often been used with great success, especially for cAMP binding proteins, and also for a cytokinin binding protein in plants (Polya and Davis, 1978). However, it is also capable of magnifying hydrophobic interactions and generating artefactual binding (see Venis, 1984, and Chapter 5.4.3). It is absolutely essential that a precipitation assay should be validated against an independent, unambiguous method. Any new binding report that relies solely on a precipitation assay should be viewed with scepticism.

2.3 AFFINITY CHROMATOGRAPHY

The basic requirement of affinity chromatography is the design of a specific adsorbent consisting of a solid support to which is covalently attached a ligand (e.g. hormone or analogue or antagonist) with high affinity for the receptor to be isolated. Ideally, if a crude mixture is passed through the adsorbent, only the receptor will be bound, contaminating proteins will pass straight through, and the pure receptor will then be recovered by changing the elution conditions. Although this ideal is seldom achieved, affinity chromatography has had many outstanding successes. The now classic paper of Cuatrecasas et al. (1968) was greatly influential in

35

stimulating interest in biospecific adsorption because it identified two important principles for successful affinity chromatography. Firstly, in addition to the basic requirements of mechanical and chemical stability during activation, coupling and operation, the support matrix should have low non-specific protein adsorption, form a loose, porous network allowing easy access to macromolecules, and retain good flow properties. It was found that these requirements were satisfied by beaded agarose gels to a very much greater degree than the cellulosic matrices used previously. Subsequently, cross-linked agaroses were found to have even better properties of chemical resistance and flow rate. Polyacrylamide beads can also be used. The second key principle was the use of a spacer arm to separate the interacting ligand from the matrix by a distance sufficient to minimise steric hindrance to macromolecule binding. Where possible, it is generally desirable to synthesize a ligand derivative with an appropriate spacer arm and then couple the derivative to the matrix. However, as the chemistry may be challenging, the alternative approach is often used, whereby the spacer is first attached to the activated matrix and the ligand is then coupled through a suitable reactive function. Details of activation, coupling and the introduction of a wide variety of reactive spacer arms suitable for the attachment of different functional residues can be found in numerous reviews (e.g. Wilchek et al., 1984) and in handbooks from commercial suppliers. The most commonly used groups for attachment purposes are $-NH_2$, $-C=O$, $-SH$ and $-OH$. Ready-activated gels and gels with a variety of reactive ligands already attached are now commercially available for 'instant' coupling and the number of ready-to-use specialist affinity adsorbents is steadily increasing. However, a suitable adsorbent for plant hormone receptors has not yet been found, although there have been several attempts to use affinity chromatography for receptor isolation in plants. These are summarized in Table 2.1 and are detailed in the appropriate Chapters. All the adsorbents (apart from those based on GA_3, for which no biological data were published) isolate selective protein fractions, but in some cases these fail to bind the hormone, while in others there are good reasons to question their receptor role. The one partial success is the matrix based on 2-hydroxy-3,5-diiodobenzoic acid (HDIBA), but its efficiency and capacity are so low (less than conventional ion exchange) that it scarcely merits the term affinity adsorbent (but see Chapter 5.1.3 for a preliminary report -

Löbler and Klämbt, 1984 - using a control spacer arm column to circumvent the low specificity). In addition to the auxin adsorbents listed in Table 2.1, six other affinity adsorbents based on different auxins, with

Table 2.1   Affinity ligands (agarose coupled) prepared for plant hormone receptor isolation (BAP = benzyladenine; i[6]Ado = isopentenyl adenosine)

Hormone class	Ligand	Spacer	Reference	Chapter
Auxins	2,4-D	Lysine	Venis (1971)	3.1
			Rizzo et al. (1977)	3.1
			Sakai and Hanagata (1983)	5.4.3
	IAA	Lysine	Roy and Biswas (1973)	5.4.1
	HDIBA	Bis oxirane	Tappeser et al. (1981)	5.1.3
Cytokinins	BAP	None	Takegami and Yoshida (1975)	6.1.2
			Reddy et al. (1983)	6.1.1
			Kharchenko et al. (1984)	3.1
	Kinetin riboside	Aminohexyl	Moore (1979)	6.1.1
	i[6]Ado	Adipic acid dihydrazide	Chen et al. (1980)	6.1.2
	BAP riboside	" "	Erion and Fox (1981)	6.1.1
	BAP	Bis oxirane	Selivankina et al. (1982a)	3.1
Gibberellins	GA$_3$	Aminoalkyl	Knöfel et al. (1975)	-

various coupling methods, have been prepared and used in attempts to purify solubilized auxin-binding proteins from maize membranes (Venis, unpublished data). There is increasing evidence (see Chapter 5.1.4) that these proteins are auxin receptors, but none of the adsorbents was able to retain the binding activity under conditions known to be optimal for auxin binding. Tappeser et al. (1981) also prepared other matrices based on hydroxy-linked analogues, but these were even less effective than their HDIBA adsorbent. It may be that effective affinity adsorbents for plant hormone receptors will yet be found, but once the initial problem of detecting any binding at all in crude preparations is solved, then with the advent of alternative rapid, high resolution purification methods in the form of FPLC (Fast Protein Liquid Chromatography), 'conventional' affinity chromatography no longer offers quite such a quantum advantage. Combined FPLC-affinity methods may be an ideal to aim for, and have been used successfully for restriction endonuclease isolation for example. Immunoaffinity chromatography has potential attractions, though desorption under native conditions can often be a problem and of course receptor isolation and antibody production are required at the outset. As will become apparent in subsequent Chapters, it is the initial problem of convincing detection of meaningful hormone binding that is of more immediate general concern than how to purify.

2.4. AFFINITY LABELLING

An affinity label - or site-directed irreversible inhibitor - is a compound that bears sufficient structural resemblance to the natural ligand to have preferential affinity for the active site over other possible binding sites, and which contains in addition a chemically reactive function capable of attaching the molecule covalently to a suitable amino acid residue in the active site region. Many chemical reagents with selectivity for different amino acid residues have been used to explore protein active sites, but usually the reagents will label suitable residues both at, and remote from, the active ligand binding site. The affinity labelling principle is an attempt to improve selectivity by incorporating the reactive group in a ligand (e.g. hormone) analogue. If the molecule is fluorescent or radioactive, its attachment can be quantitated and monitored. Thus the general structure of a chemical affinity reagent can be denoted as R-X, where R is capable of being specifically and reversibly bound to the active site, and X is a chemically reactive group.

An important variant of the general method is photoaffinity labelling, using a reagent R-P in which P is a group that is chemically unreactive in the dark, but upon irradiation with UV or near-UV light is converted to a highly reactive, species P*, with a very short half-life. P* then reacts covalently with a group in the active site before R-P* can dissociate from the site. In principle, photoaffinity labels should be more specific than 'conventional' affinity labels, since the analogue is presented to the system in the dark, allowing it first to reach the receptor site (possibly inside an intact cell) and bind non-covalently. Only then is the reactive species generated, photolytically, to react non-selectively with a variety of amino acid residues, e.g. by hydrogen abstraction or insertion into C-H bonds. Ideally, therefore, the reactive species is generated only at the active site, where it is able to react rapidly and indiscriminately with whatever groups are in the immediate vicinity. The most commonly used photoaffinity functions are diazoacyl compounds (generating carbenes), aryl azides (giving nitrenes), and $\propto$, β-unsaturated ketones (producing a diradical). A general review of photoaffinity labelling can be found in Bayley and Knowles (1977) and specific applications to (animal) hormone receptors in Linsley et al. (1981). A further refinement is photosuicide labelling (see Goeldner et al., 1982). Suicide reagents - or mechanism based irreversible inhibitors - are generally considered in relation to enzymes, whereby the normal catalytic mechanism is used to generate a reactive inhibitor species at the active site. More generally, however, any ligand that can be activated by interaction with an active site (including non-enzyme, e.g. receptor, sites) will be a suicide reagent, and if the activation is induced by light, then the process becomes one of photosuicide labelling. For example, an active site tryptophan can, after photoexcitation, undergo an energy transfer reaction with a suitable photoaffinity acceptor (e.g. aryl diazonium salts), leading to covalent attachment of the affinity label at the active site.

The fact that a putative affinity reagent labels a receptor and/or inhibits binding does not necessarily mean that the molecule reacts at the active site. If it does, then it should be possible to reduce inactivation or labelling by carrying out the reaction in the presence of the natural ligand (or analogue), and this type of experiment should always be performed as part of the affinity labelling protocol. The same principle can often be used to improve selectivity of incorporation by means of differential labelling. The strategy here is to modify first with non-radioactive reagent in the presence of a high concentration of the ligand. In this step, the receptor binding sites are protected, but other potential reactive sites are allowed to react. The ligand is then removed, and the reaction is repeated, but this time with radioactive reagent. Ideally, therefore, only the sites originally protected by the ligand should react and be labelled.

Affinity labelling can have many uses, e.g.:

1. Inferences can be drawn regarding amino acid residues in the binding site environment, based on known functional group reactivities under different conditions (see Chapter 5.1.2). Information on site geometry can be obtained by varying the substitution position of reactive groups, and by cross-linking with bifunctional reagents.

2. With radioactive or fluorescent labels, peptide sequences at the binding site can be tagged, purified and identified. With multimeric proteins, information on patterns of subunit labelling can identify those involved in binding and provide information on subunit interactions (Chapter 6.1.1).

3. Cellular localisation of receptors can be studied and changes in amount or distribution during development or differentiation evaluated.

4. It can provide a means of initially detecting a receptor (Chapter 6.3) and then facilitating its subsequent purification. With hydrophobic membrane-bound proteins, binding activity may be lost on solubilization and an affinity label (provided that it is genuinely site-specific) may provide the only means of monitoring the receptor for purification and characterization.

The Chapter sections cited above provide examples of the few cases where affinity labelling has been attempted with plant hormone-binding proteins. The most dramatic success to date has undoubtedly been the use of photoaffinity labelling to detect the presence of ABA receptors in guard cells (Hornberg and Weiler, 1984; Chapter 6.3).

3 Mediators, Messengers and Model Systems

Several reports, mainly prior to the development of unambiguous plant hormone-binding systems during the 1970s, have described factors that appeared to be implicated in hormonal effects on RNA synthesis, though hormone binding was either not examined or could not be demonstrated. To a certain extent these are only of historical interest, but it is worth considering them briefly since it may be that some of these systems should be re-examined using the more selective probes for hormone-related RNA synthesis now available (see Chapter 1). In addition this chapter will consider binding to model membranes, effects on enzyme activities in vitro, and putative second messengers.

3.1. NON-BINDING MEDIATORS

Matthysse and Phillips (1969) reported that RNA synthesis by tobacco or soybean nuclei was stimulated by addition of the auxin 2,4-D provided that 2,4-D was also present in the nuclear isolation medium. If the nuclei were sedimented from a medium lacking 2,4-D, then RNA synthesis by the nuclei was unaffected by subsequent addition of the auxin, but auxin sensitivity could be restored by adding back the supernatant fraction obtained from the nuclear centrifugation. It was inferred that, in the absence of 2,4-D, some factor required for the auxin response was lost from the nuclei. This factor, apparently protein, could be partially purified either from the nuclear lysates or from post-chromatin supernatant of pea buds. The factor was also active, in the presence of 2,4-D, in stimulating RNA synthesis by exogenous polymerase with pea bud chromatin as template, but not with purified DNA. It was claimed, though without supporting data, that the effect was an auxin-specific one on template activity. Factors prepared from different tissues of peas showed somewhat greater activity on chromatin derived from the same tissue, and there was some indirect evidence that the stimulatory factor might bind to chromatin in the presence of 2,4-D (Matthysse, 1970).

Treatment of soybean hypocotyls with 2,4-D for 4-24 hours before harvesting causes a large increase in the activity of chromatin-bound RNA polymerase (O'Brien et al., 1968), the increase being mainly in the nucleolar enzyme, polymerase I (Hardin and Cherry, 1972). A protein fraction prepared from cotyledons stimulated polymerase from control, but not from 2,4-D-treated tissue (Hardin et al., 1970). It was suggested that this protein might mediate the action of the hormone in vivo, so that polymerase from auxin-treated tissue, having been already 'activated' by the hormone-receptor complex, would be unresponsive to in vitro addition of the factor. Somewhat similarly, the activity of nucleolar RNA polymerase from lentil roots was doubled in tissue treated with IAA (Teissere et al., 1973). Fractionation of the non-histone chromosomal proteins yielded four fractions that stimulated activity of the polymerase (Teissere et al., 1975), two of which were studied in more detail and appeared to be initiation factors. It was claimed that the 'level' of one of these factors was doubled in auxin-treated tissue, though examination of the elution profiles suggests that the increase in activity was not really more than 25%. It is possible that this factor could bear some relationship to the soybean factor of Hardin et al. (1970), although the soybean protein was derived from the high-speed supernatant fraction, rather than the chromosomal pellet. A model proposed by Hardin et al. (1972) suggested that both rapid and long-term auxin responses could be mediated by a common auxin receptor in the plasma membrane. The basis of this suggestion was the finding that putative plasma membrane fractions stimulated soybean RNA polymerase and that the active factor could be released from the membranes by incubation with IAA or 2,4-D, but not by the inactive analogue 3,5-D (3,5-dichlorophenoxyacetic acid). This report bears a superficial resemblance to some of the findings of Likholat et al. (1974) for wheat coleoptiles (see Chapter 5). Subsequently it was found that the soybean factor is certainly not protein but is ethanol-soluble and of low molecular weight (Clark et al., 1976). Such a substance is unlikely to function as a receptor in the generally accepted sense, and should more appropriately be regarded as a 'stimulatory factor'.

Attempts have been made to isolate auxin receptors by affinity chromatography, using the L-lysine derivatives of 2,4-D or IAA coupled to cyanogen bromide-activated agarose (Venis, 1971). When crude supernatants prepared from pea or maize shoots were passed over such columns, small amounts of protein were retained and could be eluted by various means, typically with 1 M NaCl followed by 2mM KOH. The fractions obtained were tested for their effects on DNA-dependent RNA synthesis, supported by E. coli polymerase. The KOH fractions promoted RNA synthesis by 40-200% in different preparations, though stimulation was not dependent on the addition of auxin to the reaction mixture. Various trivial explanations for factor activity were eliminated and there was some evidence that the effect was on RNA chain initiation. To account for the lack of an auxin requirement for stimulation of RNA synthesis, it was suggested either that passage through the affinity column may transform the factor to an active configuration in which further contact with auxin is not required or that in vivo, auxin may simply permit activity to be expressed by transporting an inherently active regulatory protein from the cytoplasm to the nucleus (a model proposed by Hardin et al., 1970). Alternatively, it was proposed that a regulatory subunit might be stripped off the protein during passage through the column, as reported for affinity chromatography of cyclic AMP-dependent protein kinase (Wilchek et al., 1971). Auxin-binding activity could not be demonstrated in the stimulatory fractions. Passage through the column might have altered the configuration of the factor to one in which auxin is not bound, either by removal of a binding subunit or through inactivation of the binding site under the somewhat harsh (2 mM KOH) conditions of elution. However, unless binding activity can be reconstituted in some way or the stimulated RNA transcripts in a homologous system shown to be auxin-related, e.g. using cDNA probes, then the possibility remains that the 2,4-D-lysine adsorbent is providing no more than a combination of ion exchange and hydrophobic interaction chromatography, and therefore that the protein retained may not have any auxin-associated function.

On the other hand, auxin-binding activity was reported for a coconut protein isolated on an IAA-lysine column with NaSCN elution (Roy and Biswas, 1977). However, many reservations about this work have been expressed (see Chapter 5.4.). In addition Rizzo et al. (1977) used the 2,4-D-lysine column and preparation methods identical to those of Venis (1971) to obtain a similar though more active factor from soybean hypocotyls. DNA-dependent RNA synthesis with E. coli polymerase was stimulated two- to seven-fold by the KOH-eluted fraction. Stimulation was also observed, in the presence of 10^{-7}M 2,4-D, using soybean polymerase I, but not with polymerase II. It may be that this factor is involved in mediating the enhancement of RNA polymerase activity that follows treatment of soybeans with 2,4-D (O'Brien et al., 1968).

Matthysse and Abrams (1970) reported the preparation of a cytokinin mediator protein from the sucrose interface region obtained during purification of pea chromatin. In the presence of kinetin or zeatin, the protein stimulated RNA synthesis (10-50%) with E. coli polymerase and either pea chromatin or pea DNA as template. Stimulation was not observed when DNA from other sources was used. The effects of inactive cytokinin analogues were not described and no further reports on this system have appeared.

Kulaeva and co-workers have isolated protein fractions from barley leaves and also from pumpkin cotyledons by chromatography on a cytokinin affinity column consisting of benzyladenine (BAP) coupled to Epoxy-Sepharose (Selivankina et al., 1982 a,b; Romanko et al., 1982) or to CNBr-Sepharose (Kharchenko et al., 1984). Two fractions were eluted by a KOH gradient, though the 254/280 nm absorbance ratio of the second peak (Selivankina et al., 1982a) suggests considerable nucleic acid contamination. Neither fraction by itself affected chromatin-bound RNA polymerase activity, but each fraction stimulated activity up to 2-3-fold when BAP (10^{-6}-10^{-3}M) was added either to the assay medium or to the homogenisation medium. Stimulation was retained when the polymerase activity was solubilized from the chromatin and assayed with calf thymus DNA as template (Selivankina et al., 1982b). In a study with barley and pumpkin both homologous and heterologous chromatin-affinity protein combinations were stimulated in the presence of BAP (Romanko et al., 1982). No cytokinin other than BAP appears to have been tested in these studies, and although the BAP column fractions are referred to as 'cytokinin-binding proteins', there is as yet no evidence that they have any cytokinin-binding activity.

Pearson and Wareing (1969) found that ABA (10^{-6}M) inhibited RNA polymerase of radish cotyledon chromatin. The effect was seen only if ABA was included in the initial grinding medium, not if it was simply added to the assay mixture, suggesting perhaps the loss of an essential mediator protein during chromatin preparation (cf. Matthysse and Phillips, 1969, discussed above). Nuclei isolated from dwarf peas in the presence of 10^{-8}M GA_3 were found to be 50-80% more active in RNA synthesis than control nuclei (Johri and Varner, 1968). The RNA product also had a higher average

molecular weight and a different nearest neighbour analysis. Stimulatory
activity declined when GA_3 was added at successively later stages of the
nuclear isolation procedure, again suggesting the possible loss of a factor
required to mediate the hormonal effect. No attempts to isolate such a
factor have been reported.

3.2. INTERACTIONS WITH ARTIFICIAL MEMBRANES

The partially hydrophobic character of plant hormones long ago led to
suggestions that their action may involve partitioning into biological
membranes, altering permeability or other properties (e.g. Veldstra, 1944
a,b). Several studies, notably by Paleg and co-workers, have sought to
examine this possibility by monitoring hormonal perturbation of various
physicochemical characteristics of artificial lipid membranes in monolayer,
bilayer or liposomal systems. Thus the permeability of soybean lecithin-
sterol liposomes to both neutral (sugar) and charged (bromate) molecules was
enhanced by GA_3, but the biologically inactive GA_8 was just as effective
(Wood and Paleg, 1972). A response was also produced by IAA, though not by
kinetin. When leakage rates were examined at different temperatures, it
appeared that GA_3 lowered the phase transition temperature of the liposomal
membranes in a concentration-dependent manner over the range 0.25-2.5 mM
(Wood and Paleg, 1974). Direct interaction between GA_3 and lecithin was
detected by proton nmr spectroscopy in $CDCl_3$ (Paleg et al., 1974),
apparently a 1:1 complex involving the GA_3 carboxyl and the quaternary
ammonium headgroup. No other gibberellins were examined and the significance
of interactions in $CDCl_3$ is open to question. More recently the effect on
phase transition temperature was confirmed by Pauls et al. (1982), using
differential scanning calorimetry (dsc) and electron spin resonance (esr)
spectroscopy of liposomes prepared from defined phospholipids and varying
proportions of gibberellin. A GA_4/GA_7 mixture (74:26) was effective, whereas
GA_8 was not, in contrast to the observations of Wood and Paleg (1972) on
glucose leakage. Interactions were enhanced by conditions that minimised
charge repulsion, i.e. at low pH where the gibberellin carboxyl (pK_a ca.
4.0) is protonated, and with the zwitterionic phosphatidylcholine rather
than the anionic phosphatidylglycerol. The nature of the dsc and esr
responses suggested that the gibberellins did not complex with the
phospholipids, but rather perturbed their ordered arrangement in the bilayer

45

through a surface association.

Both Weigl (1969) and Veen (1974) observed that lecithin dissolved in CCl_4 caused IAA and other auxins to partition into the organic phase, but the later report concluded that the lecithin interaction was not correlated with biological activity. Kennedy (1971) and Kennedy and Harvey (1972) examined interactions of a range of auxins with two model membrane systems by measuring, respectively, effects on conductivity across lecithin-impregnated Millipore filters, and adsorption to lecithin and lecithin/cholesterol liposomes. With the liposomal system, changes in ion flux were also determined. In all cases, evidence was obtained of lipid interaction with the protonated forms of auxins and analogues, but effects on membrane properties required fairly high concentrations (0.1-1 mM) and did not correlate well with auxin activity. For example, adsorption of the active (+) and inactive (-) isomers of 2,4,5-trichlorophenoxy-isopropionic acid to lecithin vesicles was identical. In their nmr studies, Paleg et al. (1974) also observed IAA-lecithin interaction, with a 2:1 stoichiometry in $CDCl_3$. It was suggested that the lecithin quaternary headgroup intercalated between the planes of two indole rings and that the IAA carboxyl was not involved in the interaction. More recently, Paleg and co-workers have carried out nmr studies under somewhat more physiological conditions by examining inter-action of IAA and auxin analogues with lecithin liposomal dispersions in D_2O. The IAA-induced changes in chemical shifts of the headgroup protons were less than in $CDCl_3$, and the interaction was strongly pH-dependent, increasing at low pH with protonation of the IAA carboxyl. The stoichiometry appeared to be 1:1 with a K_d of 4.7 mM at pH 4 (Jones, G.P. et al., 1984). With a range of auxins and analogues the degree of interaction, although weak (K_d 2-10 mM for active auxins), showed a general correlation with physiological activity, the major anomaly being 2,4-D with a K_d of 66 mM (Jones and Paleg, 1984a). Interactions of IAA with different homologous series of quaternary ammonium amphiphiles showed a sharp increase at a C_8 chain length, probably attributable to micelle formation and suggesting that only weak interactions occur with less ordered lipid systems (Jones and Paleg, 1984b).

There has been one report (Stillwell and Hester, 1983) that kinetin, at concentrations exceeding 0.5 mM, increases the water permeability of liposomes prepared from both natural and synthetic phospholipids.

Benzyladenine was less effective and adenine inactive.

In all these studies it is clear that the affinities involved are generally at least 3 orders of magnitude lower than would be expected from the physiological activities of the various hormones, and that structural and enantiomeric specificity (where examined) is low. It can be expected that the lipid components of cellular membranes will have an important influence on hormone penetration and partition, and on other properties such as membrane receptor mobility. It is of interest that Erdei et al. (1979) reported that delipidation of microsomal Ca^{2+}, K^+-ATPase preparations from rice roots abolished ionic and auxin stimulation, but that these properties were restored by reconstitution with lecithin. Nevertheless, relative to proteins the limited possibilities for conformational and compositional flexibility in lipid structures make it improbable that they can function as receptors in themselves.

3.3. MODULATION OF ENZYME ACTIVITY

There have been various sporadic reports of hormone (mostly auxin) activation of enzyme activities in vitro, but generally it has not proved possible to substantiate these claims. A rather more concerted effort has been directed towards effects on ATPase activity, since activation of a membrane-bound ATPase is a requirement of the proton pump model of auxin action (see Chapter 1.3.) and would constitute a functional cell-free response coupled (presumably) to auxin-receptor interaction. For some considerable time this quest was unsuccessful, but more recently promising progress has been made.

The first report on cell-free ATPase activation was from Kasamo and Yamaki (1974), who claimed ca. 150% stimulation of a plasma membrane ATPase with 10^{-13}M IAA. The effect was essentially independent of IAA concentration over the range 10^{-13}-10^{-5}M. At 10^{-13}M IAA it was calculated (Venis, 1977a) that their reaction mixture contained not more than one molecule of IAA for every 250 ATPase molecules, which is difficult to reconcile with any significant enzyme activation. No information on auxin specificity was presented, apart from some data using crude extracts (Kasamo and Yamaki, 1973) where the effects were very small (e.g. 10% stimulation at 10^{-14}M NAA) and the only inactive compound tested was tryptamine. Erdei et al. (1979) reported up to 50% stimulation of a microsomal Ca^{2+}, K^+-ATPase from rice

47

roots by IAA or 2,4-D(10^{-10}-10^{-8}M) both in vivo and in vitro. It is not clear that this is an auxin-specific response as no physiologically inactive analogues were tested.

A somewhat more cohesive, though still tentative, picture is beginning to emerge as a result of several publications from Scherer in which membrane isolation conditions were designed to minimise phospholipase activity. Scherer and Morré (1978), working with soybean hypocotyls, examined the activity of several phosphatases in membrane fractions from sucrose gradients. The ATPase activity of one of these, thought to be enriched in plasma membrane, was stimulated by about 25% by 2,4-D at 10^{-9}M and 10^{-6}M, but not by the inactive analogue 2,3-D. Release of phosphate from an unidentified endogenous substrate was also promoted by 2,4-D (at concentrations from 10^{-9}-10^{-4}M) to a similar extent, though no other compounds were tested. Similar procedures, this time with zucchini and pumpkin hypocotyls (Scherer, 1981) yielded membrane fractions in which ATPase activity was stimulated 35-50% by 10^{-6}M IAA, provided that 10^{-4}M PAA (phenylacetic acid) was also present. Without PAA, 10^{-4}M IAA was needed for ATPase stimulation, while 10^{-8}M IAA was actually inhibitory. The effect of PAA alone was not shown, though stated to be much smaller than the auxin effects. The implication was that the enhancing influence of PAA may in some way be related to its inhibition of IAA binding to endoplasmic reticulum (ER) membranes (Dohrmann et al., 1978; see Chapter 5.1.1.). It seems unlikely that this is simply a 'sparing' phenomenon, allowing IAA to bind to plasma membrane sites, since the concentration of free IAA would not be appreciably lowered by the density of ER auxin binding sites present. The auxin effect was assigned partially to plasma membrane ATPase, though the gradient distribution of stimulated activity was very broad. It was claimed that the stimulation was auxin-specific, since (in the presence of 10^{-4}M PAA) 2,4-D was effective, but not the inactive analogues 2,3-D and 3,5-D. While the tabulated data showed this to be the case for ATPase in the 0.6-0.9M sucrose fraction, the analogues had about 60% of the activity of 2,4-D on membrane ATPase in the 1.0-1.2M sucrose region.

It now seems that one of the reasons for the difficulties encountered in obtaining reproducible auxin stimulation of ATPase activity (including a large body of unpublished data from many laboratories) has been the tendency to work at saturating (millimolar) substrate concentrations. A preliminary

48

conference report from Moloney and Pilet (1982) was the first to highlight
this problem, but the first fully-published data have come once again from
Scherer (1984 a,b). He showed that in plasma membrane-containing fractions
from zucchini hypocotyls, stimulation of ATPase by IAA and by 2,4-D
(Fig. 3.1) decreased as the ATPase concentration was raised. It was
therefore suggested that the affinity of the enzyme for ATPase was increased
in the presence of auxin, and this suggestion was supported by double
reciprocal analysis. On average, IAA reduced the apparent K_m 2.2-fold, from

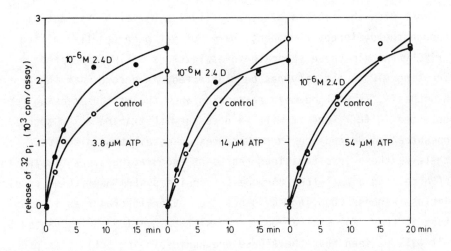

Fig. 3.1 - Stimulation of ATPase activity by 2,4-D at different
ATP concentrations (Scherer, 1984a)

ca. 0.2mM to around 0.1 mM. The auxin effects were thus most readily seen at
micromolar substrate concentrations, necessitating the use of ATP- -^{32}P; at
about 10^{-5}M ATP, the mean stimulation of initial velocity by IAA (10^{-6}M) was
ca. 30%. In both papers 2,3-D was tested as a physiologically inactive
analogue, and found to be somewhat less active than 2,4-D in stimulating
ATPase, though with a definite effect nevertheless.

These membrane fractions were also active in ATP-dependent H$^+$ transport,
as monitored by quinacrine fluorescence quenching (Scherer, 1984 a,b). It
was thought that this activity might be identical with the auxin-sensitive
ATPase, but auxin stimulation of H$^+$ transport was difficult to detect at the

low ATP concentrations (and hence low transport velocities) needed. Stimulation of electrogenic H^+ transport has, however, been claimed for pea and maize root membrane vesicles in several abstract reports (Moloney and Pilet, 1982; Moloney et al., 1983; Gabathuler et al., 1983; Gabathuler and Cleland, 1984). Hyperpolarisation was detected by ^{14}C-SCN' uptake, and the pH gradient by uptake of ^{14}C-imidazole or ^{14}C-methylamine, or by fluorescence quenching. The ATP-dependent activities were partially inhibited by orthovanadate (suggesting the presence of plasma membrane vesicles) and by a protonophore, and were stimulated by IAA (10^{-6}M) but not by benzoic acid. The K_m for ATP was reduced by IAA without affecting V_{max}, in agreement with the reports of Scherer (1984 a,b) for ATPase activity.

Although the different components have not yet been totally unified, it seems likely that in these separate investigations auxin-stimulated H^+-translocating ATPase activity has been detected, in accord with the proton pump hypothesis. It will be more reassuring when the various meeting reports are published in full, and it will be necessary to examine auxin specificity and concentration-dependence in rather greater detail than hitherto. Nevertheless, these investigations represent encouraging steps towards the goal of obtaining a cell-free hormone-responsive system permitting studies of stimulus-response coupling. Evidence from other laboratories for auxin receptors in these and similar membranes will be considered in Chapter 5, where it will be seen that the ATPase and auxin-binding activities probably reside on different proteins, but that functional association is implied by results of reconstitution experiments with bilayer lipid membranes (Thompson, M. et al., 1983). Evidence of stimulus-response coupling involving RNA synthesis (Van der Linde et al., 1984) will also be considered in the later Chapter, since this work was preceded by detailed studies of auxin binding in the same system.

3.4. SECOND MESSENGERS

Investigations on 3',5'-cyclic AMP (cAMP) in plants have passed through three distinct phases. First, following the establishment of cAMP as a mediator of the action of many peptide and catecholamine hormones and of other cellular signals in animals, and its role in bacterial gene regulation (see e.g. Robison et al., 1968), many papers in the early 1970s sought to invoke a role of cAMP as a second messenger in the action of plant hormones, particularly gibberellins and auxins. These were based on mammalian precepts, whereby the hormone binds to its receptor, leading to activation of adenylate cyclase and enhanced synthesis of cAMP which in turn binds to regulatory subunits on cAMP-dependent protein kinase. The activated kinase then phosphorylates key enzymes, modifying their activity. The enzyme responsible for removing the messenger, cAMP phosphodiesterase, is also allosterically regulated. The early flurry of plant papers therefore purported to demonstrate either an effect of the hormone on cAMP synthesis, the mimicking by applied cAMP of a hormonal response, or an effect of the hormone on cAMP degredation.

These reports suffered from various deficiencies, reviewed in detail by Lin (1974), in particular the uncritical identification of cAMP. The second phase of the cAMP story was characterised by more careful pieces of work, notably from Keates (1973) and Bressan et al. (1976), the latter report showing that plant extracts contain interfering substances that give false positives in supposedly specific biochemical assays for cAMP. Studies such as these seemed to revise estimates of putative cAMP levels in plants down to about 1% of those in resting animal cells and by the time the subject was reviewed by Amrhein (1977) the general view was that these levels, even if real, were unlikely to be of physiological relevance.

In the third phase, cAMP has regained respectability through its rigorous identification in plant tissues by GC-MS, both by Newton et al. (1980) and by Johnson et al. (1981). Whereas the former laboratory had steadfastly maintained that their earlier methods satisfactorily established the identity of cAMP (see review by Brown and Newton, 1981) it was, perhaps unfairly, the latter report, from an 'uncommitted' group, that had the greater rehabilitative influence. The levels of cAMP detected (around 100 pmol/g fresh weight) are of the same order as those found in resting mammalian cells. This cycle of events does not render the early plant work any more reliable, but it does open the way for a more careful re-examination of the possible role of cAMP as a second messenger of plant hormone action. So far (early 1985) no firm links have been established.

The second messenger currently most favoured in plants is undoubtedly calcium. Calcium has been implicated in numerous physiological processes, such as geotropism, phototropism, cell elongation, cell division, protoplasmic streaming, senescence, abscission, pollen-tube growth (Dieter,

1984). In animal cells the concentration of free cytoplasmic calcium is maintained at around 10^{-7}M or less by ATP-dependent calcium extrusion across the plasma membrane and secretion into organelles. Cellular stimulation (e.g. electrical, hormonal) raises cytoplasmic calcium to 10^{-6}-10^{-5}M by activating calcium channels in the plasma membrane and/or reducing pump activity. As a result, calcium binds to regulatory proteins, of which the most widely distributed is the heat-stable protein calmodulin (Cheung, 1980). The active calcium-calmodulin complex (K_d ca. 10^{-6}M) then in turn binds with high affinity to a number of target enzymes, causing their activation. This activation may be direct, or phosphorylation-dependent via the mediation of a calmodulin-regulated protein kinase. Inactivation is accomplished by phosphoprotein phosphatase-catalysed dephosphorylation. Not all calcium-dependent protein kinases are calmodulin regulated and other protein kinases are dependent on different divalent cations. Nevertheless, it is now apparent that the activity of both insulin and steroid hormone receptors is regulated by reversible phosphorylation-dephosphorylation and that a protein kinase is a component of the receptor itself (Garcia et al., 1983; Kasuga et al., 1983; Petruzzelli et al., 1984). Steroid receptor autophosphorylation is calcium-dependent and activity of estradiol receptor can also be modulated by a separate cytoplasmic calcium-calmodulin-dependent kinase (Auricchio et al., 1984).

In plants the chain of events is somewhat more speculative, but calmodulin or calmodulin-like activity has been found in all lower and higher plants investigated and a number of calcium-calmodulin-dependent enzymes are now known (Dieter, 1984), including NAD kinase, calcium transport ATPase, quinate:NAD oxidoreductase (QORase) and several protein kinases. The identity of the kinase substrates is for the most part unknown. One exception is QORase, which has been shown to undergo activation by calcium-calmodulin-dependent phosphorylation, and inactivation by dephosphorylation (Ranjeva et al., 1983). In addition, high affinity binding of nitrendipine, a calcium channel blocker, has been detected in pea membranes (Hetherington and Trewavas, 1984).

There is no question that calcium is a key metabolic regulator in plants, but evidence that the calcium-calmodulin system transduces hormonal signals is at present based largely on antagonism of physiological responses by phenothiazines and other calmodulin-binding drugs. Thus Elliott (1983)

reported that benzyladenine-induced synthesis of betacyanin in Amaranthus
seedlings was inhibited by phenothiazines (I_{50} 0.1-0.2 mM) and by
anaesthetic amines such as penfluridol (I_{50} 0.3-0.5 mM). When the cytokinin
effect was potentiated by red light or by the fungal toxin fusicoccin (which
exerts many auxin-like physiological responses, but more rapidly), the
calmodulin antagonists were effective at slightly lower concentrations, and
they were also somewhat more active on another cytokinin-dependent response,
soybean callus growth. In a further report (Elliott et al., 1983),
trifluoperazine (TFP) and tetracaine were used as representatives of the
phenothiazine and anaesthetic classes respectively, and found to inhibit
IAA-induced growth of wheat coleoptile sections and GA_3-induced amylase
synthesis in barley aleurones. Obata et al. (1983) also observed inhibitions
by calmodulin antagonists in the aleurone system, though only at 10^{-2}M and
only on the amylase secreted into the medium, rather than the enzyme
retained within the tissue. In contrast, Lado et al. (1981) obtained
stimulatory responses with TFP (5×10^{-5}M) and related compounds using maize
coleoptiles and other tissues, in that the antagonists enhanced growth and
H^+ secretion induced by sub-optimal concentrations of fusicoccin. It is
perhaps significant that Elliott and co-workers also observed a tendency for
slight stimulation of hormone responses at lower (ca. 10^{-5}M) TFP
concentrations. The interpretation of the different responses is not
immediately obvious, but perhaps the stimulatory effects observed at
concentrations that are better related to the I_{50} values of the drugs on
calmodulin-dependent processes in vitro are more significant than the
possibly non-specific effects obtained at higher concentrations.

The report of Erdei et al. (1979) on auxin activation of a Ca^{2+}, K^+-
ATPase in rice root microsomes was noted in the preceding section.
Subsequently the same group (Olah et al., 1983) found that treatment of
wheat seedlings in nutrient culture with 10^{-8}M benzyladenine (BAP) led to a
3-fold increase in activity of a calcium and calmodulin-dependent ATPase in
root microsomal preparations. The kinetic properties of the enzyme were
altered, the affinity towards calcium increasing nearly 6-fold and the V_{max}
by 70%. It was suggested that BAP induced new calmodulin-binding sites in
the membranes, though this was not readily apparent from the data shown.
Nor, unfortunately, was the effect of any compound other than BAP examined.
Treatment of elongating soybean hypocotyl sections with IAA for 1-2 hours

53

increased ATP-dependent Ca^{2+} accumulation in microsomal fractions by up to 100% (Kubowicz et al., 1982). It was presumed that this activity represented a Ca^{2+} efflux pump in everted plasma membrane vesicles. In contrast, zeatin treatment of similar sections inhibited Ca^{2+} transport, but with meristematic and maturing zones of the hypocotyl zeatin pretreatment promoted activity (Table 3.1). Other cytokinins were also effective, though

Table 3.1 - ATP-dependent Ca^{2+} uptake by membrane vesicles from different regions of soybean hypocotyl as affected by tissue pretreatment with IAA (10^{-5}M) or zeatin (5×10^{-5}M). Hypocotyl measurements are distances below the cotyledons (Kubowicz et al., 1982).

Pretreatment	Region of hypocotyl			
	0-5 mm	5-10 mm	10-20 mm	20-30 mm
	n mol Ca^{2+}/mg protein/30 min			
Control	8.7	12.3	13.3	6.7
IAA	7.1	16.4	23.7	7.3
Zeatin	19.3	13.6	7.4	15.7

other auxins were either inactive (2,4-D) or led to only a temporary elevation of transport activity (NAA). When added directly to the reaction medium, IAA and zeatin had little or no effect on Ca^{2+} transport, indicating that modulation of the efflux pump requires the participation of other factors or metabolic changes that are brought about by the hormone during in vivo treatment. For auxin at least, Hanson and Trewavas (1982) speculated that the missing factor is induced synthesis or activation of calmodulin, and further that the enhanced calcium efflux underlies auxin-stimulated proton efflux by releasing the H^{+}-pumping ATPase from calcium inhibition. (This inhibition might be due to Ca^{2+}-dependent phosphorylation of the ATPase; Zocchi et al., 1983). The suggestion of calmodulin involvement would be consistent with the inhibitory effects of calmodulin antagonists on auxin-induced growth referred to earlier (Elliott et al., 1983). Hanson and

Trewavas (1982) also proposed that the more rapid effects of fusicoccin arise from a more direct action on the H^+-ATPase, somehow bypassing the Ca^{2+} block. On the other hand, the stimulatory effects of TFP noted by Lado et al. (1981) would imply some involvement of calmodulin in fusicoccin action also.

Membrane vesicles prepared from soybean hypocotyls showed enhanced release of preloaded $^{45}Ca^{2+}$ in the presence of low concentrations (10^{-6}M optimum) of IAA or 2,4-D (Buckhout et al., 1981). The inactive analogue 2,3-D was either without effect or produced an opposite response, i.e. increased calcium association. The significance of the auxin effect is not clear, but is not specific to calcium, as a similar release of $^{54}Mn^{2+}$ was also observed. It was suggested that enhanced calcium release arose from the observed auxin-induced reduction in Ca^{2+}-binding sites in the membranes. The loss of these sites was subsequently attributed to auxin-enhanced turnover of membrane phosphatidylinositol (Morré et al., 1984), though there did not seem to be any clear parallels with the diglyceride-inositol triphosphate control cycles of mammalian cells (Berridge and Irvine, 1984). Auxin-stimulated ^{45}Ca release has also been noted with soybean protoplasts, in a preliminary report from Cohen and Lilly (1984). Inhibition of ^{45}Ca uptake was also observed, and the effect was specific to active auxins (IAA, NAA, 2,4-D), while compounds with little or no physiologically activity (benzoic acid, 2-NAA) were without effect. The system appears to have some of the characteristics of an auxin-regulated Ca^{2+} channel and it may be that the observations of Buckhout et al. (1981) are better interpreted similarly, rather than as release from binding sites.

There are several reports of protein phosphorylation modulated by plant hormones in vivo (e.g. Chapman et al., 1975; Murray and Key, 1978). More recently (Morré et al., 1984) slight in vitro stimulation of protein phosphorylation in soybean membranes was observed with 10^{-6}M 2,4-D. However, the effect was not statistically significant and was inhibited, not enhanced, by calcium. The notion that receptor activity may be regulated by phosphorylation-dephosphorylation, as for mammalian hormone receptors, is an attractive one, and there are preliminary indications that receptors for both fusicoccin and auxin may be so regulated (see Chapter 5.4.2.). Whether calcium is involved in these systems is not yet known. At present the clearest evidence for phosphorylation of a hormone-binding protein in plant material is the cytokinin-binding protein (CBP) of wheat germ, which is phosphorylated by a calcium-independent protein kinase from the same source (Polya and Davies, 1983). Unfortunately, the general characteristics of CBP do not encourage the view that it is a hormone receptor (see Chapter 6).

Clearly, the general evidence for mediation of plant hormone action by calcium and/or by protein phosphorylation is somewhat nebulous at present. However, as the various metabolic functions of cytoplasmic calcium in plants become clarified further, it will be surprising if connections with hormone action are not more firmly established.

Recently, connections have been established in mammalian systems between calcium mediation and the action of another well-investigated group of possible cellular messengers, the polyamines, and it seems possible that changes in polyamine concentrations may even precede and determine altered Ca^{2+} fluxes. Polyamines, such as spermine, spermidine and putrescine, are present in cells at up to millimolar concentrations and display varied biological activities, including stimulation of DNA replication, transcription, and of mRNA translation. Elevated polyamine concentrations and enhanced activity of ornithine decarboxylase (ODC), a key regulatory enzyme in their biosynthesis, are among the earliest events associated with cell proliferation and differentiation. It has been found (Qi et al., 1983) that polyamines, particularly spermine, will selectively inhibit both phospholipid-regulated and calmodulin-regulated calcium-dependent protein kinases of mammalian origin, without affecting c-AMP- or c-GMP-dependent protein kinases. This suggests that spermine and calcium may interact in regulation of protein phosphorylation. More pertinently, Koenig et al. (1983) discovered that the early (within 1 min.) responses to testosterone stimulation in mouse kidney cortex, which include increased Ca^{2+} fluxes and mobilisation of intracellular calcium, are dependent upon an even more rapid, transient increase in ODC activity and a sustained increase in polyamine content. It was proposed that binding of testosterone to its receptor activates (possibly by reversible phosphorylation) a latent ODC located in or near the plasma membrane. The synthesized polyamines then generate the Ca^{2+} signal by cation exchange displacement of bound calcium from the plasma membrane (thereby opening calcium gates) and from organelles. While detailed elements of the model are somewhat speculative, the experimental evidence nevertheless pointed clearly to a key role for polyamines in transduction of a receptor-mediated signal.

In plants too there is heightened interest in the possible second messenger role of polyamines, though clear connections with signal transduction are not firmly established. Polyamines have been implicated in many physiological processes, including responses to hormone application, and various developmental changes under endogenous hormone control such as somatic embryogenesis (Bradley et al., 1984; Feirer et al., 1984) and floral development (Malmberg and McIndoo, 1983). The first link between plant hormones and polyamines came from the work of Bagni and co-workers starting in the 1960s (reviewed in Bagni et al., 1982) showing that auxin-induced growth of Jerusalem artichoke tuber explants is associated with a several-fold increase in polyamine levels within 1 hour, and that polyamines can largely replace the auxin requirement for growth. This system probably still represents one of the clearest links between polyamines and hormone action in plants, though connections of one sort or another have since been established with all the plant hormones, particularly gibberellic acid (e.g. Dai et al., 1982; Kyriakidis, 1983). Galston especially has of recent years been a vigorous advocate of polyamines as second messengers in transmitting cellular stimuli of various kinds - hormonal, light and stress (e.g. Galston, 1983). While it is certainly established that polyamines can exert important regulatory effects in plants, it is not yet clear that changes in polyamine metabolism flow directly from cellular stimulation rather than being independent events accompanying other metabolic change. For example, Lin (1984) could find no changes in polyamine metabolism during the 8-hour lag period of GA_3-induced amylase synthesis in barley aleurones and concluded that polyamines did not serve as second messengers of gibberellin action in this system. If, however, polyamine biosynthesis was inhibited during the imbibition period prior to GA_3 addition, then subsequent GA_3-induced enzyme synthesis was substantially reduced, suggesting that the establishment of a minimum polyamine level in the tissue was in some way a necessary though insufficient condition for enzyme induction. Evidently the precise roles of polyamines and their relationships to plant hormone action requires considerable further investigation before any conclusions as to participation in receptor-response coupling can be reached. Protein phosphorylation is an important mechanism in mediating other cellular signals and merits investigation in relation to hormone-polyamine

57

interaction in plants. Stimulation of Mg^{2+}-dependent protein phosphorylation by polyamines, particularly spermine, has in fact been demonstrated in maize (Veluthambi and Poovaiah, 1984) and the spectrum of phosphorylated proteins was distinct from that induced by Ca^{2+}. Hormonal regulation in this system awaits exploration.

4 Binding Sites for Auxin Transport Inhibitors

Early attempts to detect auxin binding to membrane fractions were unsuccessful, so attention was directed instead towards binding of the synthetic auxin transport inhibitor N-1-naphthylphthalamic acid, NPA (Fig. 4.3) which could be prepared tritiated at high specific activity. In some respects the NPA binding sites now represent the best studied receptor system in plants; in particular the sites have been localised immunochemically and their role clearly involves auxin transport, even if their precise function remains to be defined.

In the original report (Lembi et al., 1971), membrane fractions from maize coleoptiles were fractionated on sucrose gradients and their ability to bind NPA-^{3}H was assayed by a pelleting technique. Binding was correlated with plasma membrane content of the fractions as assessed by phospho-tungstate-chromate (PTC) staining, a method supposedly specific for plasmalemma (though this is questioned, see e.g. Quail and Browning, 1977; Hall, 1983). Binding was reversible and of high affinity, with an approximate K_d of 2×10^{-8}M. A plasmalemma localization was also subsequently suggested on the basis of correlation of binding and glucan synthetase II activities on sucrose gradients (Normand et al., 1975; Ray, 1977). No displacement of bound NPA-^{3}H was obtained with auxins (IAA, NAA, 2,4-D), other hormones (GA$_3$, abscisic acid) or with 10^{-5}M 2,3,5-triiodo-benzoic acid (TIBA), a chemically distinct auxin transport inhibitor which is itself an auxin analogue (Lembi et al., 1971; Thomson, 1972). The binding affinity of NPA was reasonably well correlated with the saturation kinetics of its effect on auxin transport (Thomson et al., 1973), though it should be noted that published affinities vary somewhat, and that some laboratories report two kinetically distinct classes of binding site (Table 4.1). The most detailed kinetic characterization has been that of Trillmich and Michalke (1979), who measured binding in the membrane suspensions both by the usual equilibrium method (centrifugation) and by following the time course of association and dissociation with a membrane filtration technique. The K_d values derived either from the ratio of the rate constants or obtained directly from the equilibrium assay were in good agreement, confirming that the interaction is a straightforward one, described by:

$$NPA + R \underset{k_{-1}}{\overset{k_1}{\rightleftharpoons}} NPA\text{-}R$$

Table 4.1   Reported affinities of NPA binding sites in maize coleoptiles

$K_d(\times 10^{-7}M)$	n,pmol/g	Reference
0.2	Not reported	Lembi et al., 1971
0.13	2	Thomson, 1972
2.2	20	
1.8	5	Normand et al., 1975
0.3	8	Trillmich and Michalke, 1979
1.0	5	Sussman and Gardner, 1980
5.0	15	
0.6	Not reported	Katekar et al., 1981

A similar conclusion was reached more recently by Maan et al. (1985a), who detected NPA binding sites in membranes from tobacco cell suspension cultures. The mean K_d value from the two independent methods was $3 \times 10^{-9}M$, an affinity about ten times greater than that observed in maize (Table 4.1). Auxins competed with NPA-^{3}H to some extent, but with very much lower affinity, e.g. over five orders of magnitude lower for IAA.

Sussman and Gardner (1980) showed that the maize binding sites could be solubilized from the membranes using the non-ionic detergent Triton X-100, yielding preparations with NPA binding kinetics very similar to those seen in the native state. Binding is not, therefore, attributable to uptake into sealed vesicles. Biphasic Scatchard plots were observed with both membrane-bound and soluble preparations and hence two populations of binding sites were suggested (Table 4.1). However, these data were obtained using a non-equilibrium gel filtration assay that required about 7 min. from application of sample to complete elution of void volume. As this is close to the $t_{0.5}$ for the complex at 0°C (Trillmich and Michalke, 1979), the non-linearity of the Scatchard plot may simply reflect heterogeneity in the dissociation state of the complex between the beginning and end of the voided volume. The solubilized sites were far more heat labile than the membranous sites and had a lower pH optimum for binding (pH 4.0 versus pH 5.0). In either state, binding activity was trypsin sensitive. The most significant change in properties upon solubilization was the ability of IAA (10^{-6}-10^{-5}M) to displace NPA-^{3}H from the binding sites, whereas with intact membranes, in agreement with earlier reports, no interaction with IAA was observed even at 0.5mM. The affinity for NAA was also enhanced, by at least an order of magnitude. This report was the first indication that the NPA binding site complex is able to interact to some degree with auxins, albeit with relatively low affinity, presumably via a region that is not accessible in the isolated membrane fragments.

Although Thomson (1972) did not detect competition by 10^{-5}M TIBA for NPA binding in maize coleoptile membranes, others subsequently found about 50% displacement of bound NPA-^{3}H by TIBA at 10^{-5}M (Depta et al., 1983; Katekar, 1985) or 10^{-4}M (Sussman and Goldsmith, 1981). Nevertheless, this order of binding affinity has been considered to be too low to account for the activity of TIBA on polar transport (I_{50} ca. 2-3 x 10^{-6}M; Thomson et al., 1973; Depta et al., 1983) and it has therefore been suggested that NPA and TIBA inhibit transport at different binding sites. Since TIBA itself moves in the polar auxin transport system (Thomson et al., 1973) and also, unlike NPA, competes effectively for auxin binding sites (K_i ca. 2 x 10^{-6}M, Batt et al., 1976, see Chapter 5), it might interact directly with auxin channels in inhibiting transport. Against this possibility, there is some evidence that the transport inhibition is non-competitive, leading Depta et al. (1983) to propose an auxin transport complex consisting of an auxin translocation site plus two distinct regulatory sites with differential affinities for NPA and for TIBA. On chemical grounds, one would certainly anticipate that NPA and TIBA should act at different sites, but existing evidence for a separate regulatory TIBA site (Depta et al., 1983) is far from clear-cut. In summary, there is little doubt that the NPA binding site is distinct from the site of auxin translocation, though the two must be in close association, e.g. as sub-units of a complex. It is also likely that TIBA and NPA act at different

61

sites, but whether the TIBA site is the auxin channel itself or a separate
regulatory site has not been resolved.

Many other compounds do in fact bind at the NPA site itself. Firstly,
several NPA derivatives were found to displace NPA-^{3}H from the maize binding
sites (Thomson and Leopold, 1974) in a manner that was approximately
compatible with their relative activities as transport inhibitors, and more
recently Katekar (1985) has reported an excellent correlation between
binding affinities of a series of arylphthalamic acids and their ability to
inhibit root gravitropism (Fig. 4.1). Thomson and Leopold (1974) also found
that NPA binding was displaceable by various morphactins, another group of

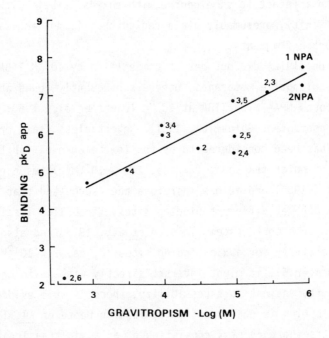

Fig. 4.1 - Correlation of receptor binding affinity and root
gravitropic activity on cress seedlings of arylphthalamic acids.
Numbers represent the chlorine substitution pattern
on phenylphthalamic acid

synthetic auxin transport inhibitors. The interaction of one of these,
chlorflurenol, was shown to be competitive by double reciprocal analysis,

with an affinity similar to that of NPA (K_i = 2.9 x 10^{-7}M). Following the demonstration by Katekar and Geissler (1975) that fluorescein and related compounds such as eosin and mercurochrome were inhibitors of auxin transport, these compounds were also shown to compete for NPA binding sites (Venis, 1981; Sussman and Goldsmith, 1981). This is illustrated in Fig. 4.2, which also demonstrates the very weak interactions of auxins and TIBA and confirms the high affinity of chlorflurenol (the morphactin used) for the NPA site.

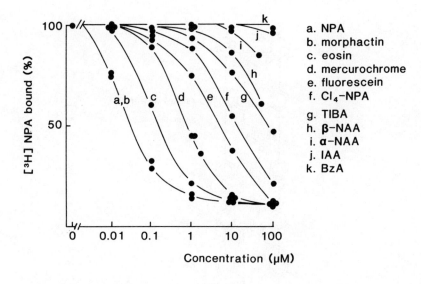

a. NPA
b. morphactin
c. eosin
d. mercurochrome
e. fluorescein
f. Cl_4-NPA
g. TIBA
h. β-NAA
i. α-NAA
j. IAA
k. BzA

Fig. 4.2 - Competition by auxin transport inhibitors, auxins and benzoic acid (B_zA) for NPA-^{3}H binding to maize membranes (Sussman and Goldsmith, 1981)

In a series of papers, Katekar has investigated in some detail the biological activities of several different classes of auxin transport inhibitor, their structure-activity relationships, and their binding affinities for the NPA receptor. Some of these structures are shown in Fig. 4.3. The structural requirements for inhibition of root geotropism (Katekar, 1976) were found to be very similar to those for inhibition of auxin transport (Katekar and Geissler, 1977). In summary, the essential features were considered to be a 2-carboxyphenyl group separated by a conjugated system of atoms from a second aromatic ring. High activity is obtained when the distance between the centres of the two extreme aromatic rings is at least 0.73 nm. Substituents on the non-carboxylated ring have little effect except insofar as they help to achieve this minimum molecular size. Thus fluorescein, which is below the critical size (Fig. 4.3) is less active than the brominated derivative eosin (Fig. 4.3 and Katekar and Geissler, 1975). Subsequently a conformational requirement was added, such that the aromatic ring bearing the carboxyl group should be out of plane

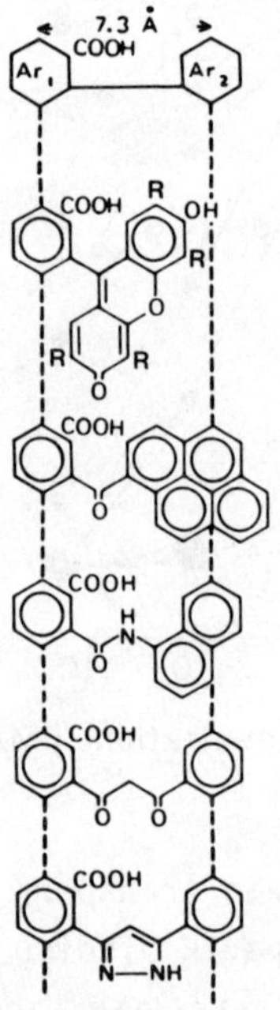

Fig. 4.3 - Structures of some phytotropin auxin transport inhibitors
(from Katekar et al., 1981)

with the rest of the molecule. The carboxyl group itself does not have to be coplanar with its ring (Katekar and Geissler, 1981). More recently (Katekar, 1985) these requirements have been considered in terms of an approximate receptor model. As well as inhibiting geotropism, the compounds under consideration also inhibit stem phototropism and elicit typical biphasic dose-response curves for inhibition of cress root growth (Katekar and Geissler, 1980). These authors proposed the term 'phytotropin' to describe this group of compounds with common molecular features and an apparently similar mode of action, and the term has gained general acceptance.

The affinity of the fluorescein group of compounds for the NPA receptor has already been noted. Katekar et al. (1981) extended these observations to include representatives of all eight chemical types of phytotropin recognised, comparing their biological activities with their effectiveness in displacing NPA-^{3}H from its binding site. Some of these data are summarised in Table 4.2, which shows that the different chemical classes do

Table 4.2   Apparent dissociation constants of binding of some phytotropins and comparison with biological activities (from Katekar et al., 1981)

Compound	K_d app.[1]	Auxin transport[2]	Root geotropism[3]
Fluorescein	7.9×10^{-6}	95	10^{-4}
PBA	6.3×10^{-8}	24	10^{-9}
NPA	6.3×10^{-8}	30	10^{-6}
CPD	1.8×10^{-7}	32	3×10^{-8}
CPP	5.0×10^{-8}	16	10^{-7}

[1] Molar concentration giving 50% reduction of specific NPA-^{3}H binding
[2] % transport at 10^{-7}M compound
[3] lowest concentration (molar) at which root georesponse is abolished

indeed bind to the same site with high affinity and in reasonable agreement with their biological activities. PBA, 2-(1-pyrenoyl) benzoic acid, is the most active phytotropin yet identified. These comparisons have since been extended to many more representatives, with excellent correlations between binding affinity and root geotropic activity, save for a few exceptions, one of which is NPA, whose biological activity is lower than might be anticipated (Katekar, 1985). However, NPA falls on the same correlation curve as the chemically related series of phenylphthalamic acids (Fig. 4.1), indicating that these compounds are systematically different in some way.

Since they are amides, it was suggested that the common feature leading to reduced biological activity is susceptibility to hydrolytic inactivation in the plant.

Katekar and Geissler (1977, 1980) did not consider morphactins to be phytotropins because they do not conform to the specified structural requirements and because they induce characteristic morphological responses of their own. It was suggested that their biological activity might derive from breakdown in the plant to 2-phenylbenzoic acids, which do fulfil the chemical requirements. However, morphactins do induce characteristic phytotropin responses, including biphasic inhibition of root growth (Katekar and Geissler, 1980), and they compete with high affinity for NPA binding in vitro (e.g. Fig. 4.2) under conditions where there is little or no possibility of such chemical transformation. They must, therefore, be conformationally compatible with the active binding site, and it seems reasonable to regard them as members of the phytotropin class and to suggest that the structural specifications of this class need to be refined.

Whatever the normal function of the NPA binding site, it is clear that it must be physically in close association with the site of auxin transport. One of the propositions of the chemiosmotic model of auxin transport, which will be considered further in the next Chapter, is that polarity of transport is achieved by efflux of auxin anions from the cell via specific, saturable anion efflux carriers that are located in the plasma membrane preferentially at the basal ends of transporting cells (Rubery and Sheldrake, 1974). Inhibitors of auxin transport (TIBA and phytotropins) are considered to act by blocking the auxin efflux carrier (Sussman and Goldsmith, 1981). On an operational basis, therefore, NPA binding should be a marker for the efflux carrier, and it is this principle that was used by Jacobs and Gilbert (1983) to localize the presumptive carriers immunochemically by means of monoclonal antibodies directed against the NPA receptor. These were produced by immunization with a crude pea membrane preparation, using inhibition of NPA binding as the selection assay. Inhibitory supernatants were incubated with median longitudinal sections of etiolated pea third internode tissue, and bound antibody was located with fluorescein-labelled rabbit anti-mouse second antibody. The published color photomicrographs showed very elegantly that the fluorescent label was associated only with parenchyma cells surrounding vascular bundles and, more

importantly, that the label was confined to U-shaped regions at the basal
ends of the cells. In plasmolyzed cells, the fluorescence remained
associated with the plasma membrane as it pulled away from the cell wall.
Using Triton-solubilized pea membrane preparations, Jacobs and Gilbert
(1983) found, as Sussman and Gardner (1980) had done in maize, that

Table 4.3   Comparison of the effects of active and inactive antibodies on
             specific and IAA-sensitive NPA binding to solubilized pea
             membranes (Jacobs and Gilbert, 1983; copyright 1983 by the AAAS)

Treatment	Radioactivity (cpm)		
	$[^3H]$NPA bound	Specific NPA binding (A - B)	IAA-sensitive NPA binding (A - C)
Inactive supernatant			
A. 10^{-9}M $[^3H]$NPA	1704		
B. 10^{-9}M $[^3H]$NPA plus 10^{-5}M NPA	952	752	526
C. 10^{-9}M $[^3H]$NPA plus 10^{-5}M IAA	1178		
Active supernatant			
A. 10^{-9}M $[^3H]$NPA	1494		
B. 10^{-9}M $[^3H]$NPA plus 10^{-5}M NPA	1141	353	-120
C. 10^{-9}M $[^3H]$NPA plus 10^{-5}M IAA	1614		

solubilization conferred IAA-sensitivity on the NPA binding sites. Moreover,
both saturable NPA binding and the IAA-sensitive component were inhibited by
antibodies from an active clone (Table 4.3). This indicated that the NPA
binding site recognized by the antibody can also interact with IAA and
therefore supports the immunofluorescence evidence in suggesting that auxin
efflux carriers are indeed preferentially located at the base of
transporting cells, as required by the chemiosmotic hypothesis. This work
constitutes the first localization of a receptor in plants and was the first
report using monoclonal antibodies to label plant tissue.

What, if anything, normally binds to the phytotropin receptor and what is the receptor's function? Both Thomson (1972) and later Katekar and Geissler (1980) have suggested that there may be an as yet unidentified natural agonist, or native phytotropin. This is certainly a reasonable expectation and has an excellent precedent in the recognition of opiate receptors long before the natural ligands (endorphins) were discovered. Hertel and co-workers (Hertel et al., 1976) have reported briefly on a solvent-extractable fraction from potatoes ('Kartoffelfaktor', or KF) that competes for NPA-^{3}H binding and inhibits auxin transport. However, this work has never been fully published and investigations in other laboratories have suggested that KF activity is associated with a complex mixture of substances, possibly long-chain fatty acids, rather than with a single, highly active substance (Venis, Sittingbourne; Gardner, Modesto; unpublished data). So, while there may very well be a natural phytotropin, it has not yet been identified. The ability of synthetic phytotropins to inhibit both auxin transport and the root geotropic response might suggest that an endogenous ligand binding to a regulatory site ('NPA receptor') on the auxin efflux carrier could play a role in the organ's response to gravity, by effecting auxin asymmetry, in accordance with the Cholodny-Went model. The U-shaped distribution of NPA sites observed immunochemically (Jacobs and Gilbert, 1983) affords the possibility of a lateral component to carrier-mediated auxin transport. On the other hand, the traditional view of the basis of geotropic curvatures has been questioned (Firn and Digby, 1980) and using immunochemical assays Mertens and Weiler (1983) were unable to detect asymmetry of auxin distribution in any gravireacting organ other than the maize coleoptile. The latter authors considered that the gravitropic response may yet be auxin-controlled, by changes in compartmentation between physiologically inactive and active pools, and it is possible that this is in some way controlled by the phytotropin site. However, as noted by Katekar (1985), the phenomena observed with synthetic phytotropins (transport and geotropic inhibition) may in fact be a wholly inadequate reflection of the true physiological role of the hypothetical endogenous ligand.

5 Binding Sites for Auxins

5.1. MEMBRANE-BOUND SITES IN MAIZE

5.1.1 General properties

The methods used originally to demonstrate NPA binding to maize coleoptile membranes (Lembi et al., 1971) were soon successful in detecting auxin binding in the same source material (Hertel et al., 1972). These pioneering papers were greatly influential in stimulating plant receptor research in several laboratories and the maize system has been particularly. well investigated, though more recently, as will be seen, zucchini membranes have proved advantageous for studying auxin transport sites.

Hertel et al. (1972), in their initial report, detected saturable binding of NAA-^{14}C and IAA-^{3}H to heterogeneous membrane preparations from maize coleoptiles. Binding was reversible and equilibrium rapid (within a few minutes at 0°C). Radioactive NAA in the pellets could be displaced by unlabelled auxins such as IAA and 2,4-D, also by TIBA, but not by the inactive compound, benzoic acid. Abscisic acid, GA_3, and NPA also failed to interact with the binding sites. The dissociation constants were estimated as 1-2 x 10^{-6}M for NAA and 3-4 x 10^{-6}M for IAA. Binding activity was destroyed by heating or by treatment with sodium lauryl sulphate, and could be largely separated from nuclear and mitochondrial markers. The same system was investigated further by Normand et al. (1975), who obtained a K_d for NAA of 1.66 x 10^{-6}M and showed that maximum NAA binding was associated with membranes, possibly endoplasmic reticulum (ER), that band on sucrose gradients at a lower density than the NPA-binding peak. Changes in the original procedure, in particular prior separation of the membranes from the supernatant by pelleting and re-suspension, yielded improved binding data and a revised K_d for NAA of 5 x 10^{-7}M (Hertel, 1974, described more fully in Ray et al. (1977a).

Investigating binding of NAA-^{14}C in greater detail over a more restricted concentration range, Batt et al. (1976) obtained data that yielded a biphasic Scatchard plot (Fig. 5.1), suggesting the presence within the membrane preparation of at least two sets of high affinity binding sites for

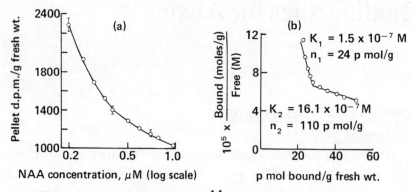

Fig. 5.1 - Binding of NAA-^{14}C by maize membranes
(a) displacement of NAA-^{14}C in membrane pellets by unlabelled NAA
(b) Scatchard-Hunston analysis of the data (Batt et al., 1976)

NAA, with dissociation constants of 1.5×10^{-7}M (site 1) and 1.6×10^{-6}M (site 2). IAA-^{14}C also appeared to bind to two sets of sites ($K_1 = 1.7 \times 10^{-6}$M; $K_2 = 5.8 \times 10^{-6}$M), whose concentrations were in good agreement with those deduced for NAA. The binding specificity of each class of sites was examined by double reciprocal analysis of NAA-binding curves performed in the presence or absence of a fixed concentration of a given auxin analogue. From many such experiments with a range of analogues it was found that all compounds tested, including inactive analogues such as benzoic acid, showed some competition with NAA for site 1 binding. Site 2 on the other hand exhibited binding specificity more compatible with the expected properties of an auxin receptor, in that only active auxins or anti-auxins were able to compete with NAA for the binding sites. The K_i values for IAA were very similar to the K_d values obtained directly from IAA-^{14}C binding, indicating that the competitive interactions studied do indeed represent competition for common classes of binding sites; a similar conclusion was reached by Ray et al. (1977b). The transport inhibitors TIBA and NPA were both found to interact with the NAA binding sites (Batt et al., 1976), but TIBA, which also has both auxin and anti-auxin properties, competed much more effectively than NPA, particularly for site 2. Nearly 90% of the total NAA-^{14}C binding activity was recovered in membrane preparations solubilized with the detergent Triton X-100, indicating that the major portion of the binding does not consist of transport into sealed vesicles.

Following differential centrifugation of the membrane preparation, the
4,000-10,000 g fraction appeared to contain a single population of NAA-
binding sites (linear Scatchard plot) with a K_d of 1.6 x 10^{-6}M,
characteristic of site 2, the auxin-specific site, whereas the 10,000-
38,000 g fraction still yielded a biphasic Scatchard plot (Batt and Venis,
1976). When the total membrane preparation (4,000-38,000 g) was fractionated
on discontinuous sucrose gradients into two bands, linear Scatchard plots
were obtained for NAA-^{14}C binding to the resolved fractions, suggesting that
one distinct set of binding sites predominated in each band. The
dissociation constants (3.8 x 10^{-7}M for the light band, 1.2 x 10^{-6}M for the
heavy band), were in reasonable agreement with those determined for site 1
and site 2 respectively in unfractionated membrane preparations, implying
that substantial resolution of the binding sites had been obtained. The
binding specificities of the two membrane bands (examined by competition
with IAA, TIBA and benzoic acid) were also compatible with this conclusion.
Analysis of binding activities and enzymic and chemical markers in membrane
fractions from multi-step sucrose gradients together with PTC staining and
electron microscopy, suggested that site 1 is located on ER or Golgi
membranes, while site 2 is associated with plasma membrane fractions.

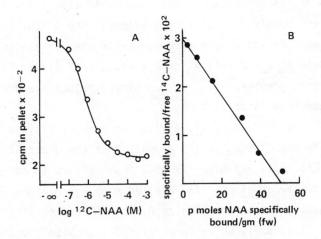

Fig. 5.2 - A. Effect of unlabelled NAA on NAA-^{14}C binding by
maize membranes. B. Scatchard plot (Ray et al., 1977a)

Ray et al. (1977a) obtained linear Scatchard plots for NAA-^{14}C binding, indicating a single kinetic class of binding sites, with a K_d of 5-7 x 10^{-7}M (Fig. 5.2). Both Normand et al. (1975) and Ray (1977) concluded, from sucrose gradient fractionation, that the majority of the NAA sites are located on ER, clearly separable from the NPA binding peak at higher density. Ray (1977) used higher resolution continuous isopycnic gradients and found that both NAA binding and ER marker enzyme peaks shifted down the gradient when 3 mM Mg^{2+} was included to prevent stripping of ribosomes from the ER. On the other hand, the NAA binding region under low Mg^{2+} conditions clearly extended into denser gradient regions essentially devoid of ER and it was concluded that a minority of the sites may be located on Golgi and/or plasma membranes. Moreover, Dohrmann et al. (1978) have reported evidence for three types of auxin-binding sites in maize membranes, based on the differential affinities of sucrose gradient fractions for different auxin analogues. These were designated site I (associated with ER), site II (suggested location on tonoplast membranes and distinguished by low affinity for the weak auxins, 2-naphthylacetic acid and phenylacetic acid, PAA) and site III, found in plasma membrane fractions and characterized by preferential binding of 2,4-D. Sites I and II could be distinguished kinetically, either by assaying in the presence (site II) or absence (site I) of PAA or, as described by Batt and Venis (1976), by assaying membrane fractions resolved on sucrose gradients. The affinities of NAA for sites I and II were in reasonable agreement with the values for the sites designated by Batt et al. (1976) as site 1 and site 2 (Table 5.1). Site III has been studied in greater detail in zucchini hypocotyls and will be discussed further in a later section.

The data analysis of Batt et al. (1976) has been criticized by Ray et al. (1977a) and by Murphy (1980a) on the grounds that the apparent site heterogeneity (Fig. 5.1) may have resulted from failure to correct for non-specific binding. Ray et al. (1977a) applied such corrections by subtracting values of residual binding remaining at 0.1 mM NAA and obtained linear Scatchard plots (Fig. 5.2), while Murphy (1980a) applied computer curve fitting procedures using binding models of varying complexity and concluded that the most reliable fit to the experimental data was obtained with a single kinetic class of binding sites (Table 5.1) plus non-specific binding. It was also shown (Murphy, 1980a) that apparently divergent K_d values in

Table 5.1 Summary of reported auxin-binding sites in maize coleoptile
membranes (PM = plasma membrane)

K_d for NAA, $\times 10^{-6}$M	No. of binding sites, pmol/g	Suggested location	Reference
1-2*	~ 50	Not examined	Hertel et al. (1972)
1.66*	14	ER	Normand et al. (1975)
0.15 (site 1)	25-30	ER/Golgi	Batt et al. (1976)
1.60 (site 2)	100-120	PM	
0.5-0.7	30-50	Mainly ER, also Golgi and/or PM	Ray et al. (1977 a,b)
0.4 (site I)	40	ER	
1.3 (site II)	20	Tonoplast	Dohrmann et al. (1978)
>5 (site III)	40	PM	
0.15	48	Not examined	Murphy (1980a)
0.35	18[/]	Not examined	Jones et al. (1984a)
9.0	164[/]		

* These data were obtained with low speed supernatants; later studies used
resuspended membrane pellets

[/] Data given as pmol/mg protein; but 1 g fresh weight contains ca. 1 mg
microsomal protein

separated membrane fractions, as observed by Batt and Venis (1976), could
arise from varying proportions of non-specific binding contributions to
kinetically comparable binding site populations.

It is certainly true that omitting such corrections will bias the kinetic
parameters obtained. On the other hand, as Rubery (1981) has observed,
subtraction of non-specific binding values from the data shown in Fig. 5.1
still does not result in linear Scatchard plots, and the extent to which
site heterogeneity is recognizable kinetically will vary according to the
balance between sites of differing affinity. Moreover, Dohrmann et al.
(1978) did correct for non-specific binding, yet still found kinetically
distinct sites both in unfractionated membranes (Table 5.1) and in resolved

'light' (NAA K_d = 6 x 10^{-7}M) and 'heavy' (K_d = 2.7 x 10^{-6}M) membrane fractions. In addition, these authors distinguished their site II from site I by a greater binding selectivity for active auxins and by lower sensitivity to inhibition by dithioerythritol and by a supernatant factor, SF, whose properties will be discussed later. (Batt et al., 1976, reached a similar conclusion with regard to the differential supernatant effect). More recently, Jones et al. (1984a) have also analysed two sets of binding sites from Scatchard plots after subtraction of non-specific binding (Table 5.1), though the alternative possibility of negative cooperativity of one class of sites was also noted.

In summary, there is little doubt that auxin-binding sites are located on more than one type of cellular membrane. The properties of sites 1 and 2 seem to approximate to those of sites I and II (Table 5.1) in terms of kinetics and specificity and there is general agreement that one class of binding site is associated with ER, while various membranes of greater buoyant density, probably including the plasma membrane, also have auxin-binding activity. What is less clear is that the sites are necessarily distinguishable kinetically, and at times it will be more convenient to discuss them as a homogeneous population. Apart from differences in the proportions of the membrane sites, at least one other potential source of inter-laboratory variation resides in the concentration of SF, which appears to reduce the affinity of the ER site for NAA (Dohrmann et al., 1978) and whose concentration varies even between different batches of the same maize cultivar (Batt et al., 1976). Both Venis (1977a) and Dohrmann et al. (1978) have suggested that the ER site could be a precursor of site 2/II. Alternatively, or additionally, if higher specificity, lower affinity binding sites of the site 2 type do in fact reside in the plasma membrane, then these could function as primary auxin discriminators and mediate an auxin-specific membrane response. Higher affinity ER sites might then accept auxin translocated from site 2 and transmit the auxin signal to the nucleus; on this basis the ER sites could be of lesser selectivity (Stoddart and Venis, 1980). Ray (1977) has suggested that the somewhat slower effects of auxins on extension growth and proton extrusion (relative to fusicoccin) would be compatible with initiation of auxin action at the ER, leading to proton movement into ER vesicles and their channeling to the cell surface. However, this proposal has been questioned (Cleland, 1982), mainly on the

74

grounds that the capacity of such a system would be inadequate to generate the proton flux required.

Binding specifity has been examined in greatest detail by Ray et al. (1977b), Dohrmann et al. (1978) and by Murphy (1980a), all of whom determined NAA-^{14}C displacement curves with a wide range of auxin analogues. There is a reasonable, though imperfect, correlation between biological activity and apparent K_d values, one of the major discrepancies being the relatively low binding affinity for highly active phenoxyacetic acids such as 2,4-D. Ray et al. (1977b) have pointed to the metabolic stability of 2,4-D relative to IAA as a possible factor offsetting low receptor affinity, and indeed in short-term (2 hour) tests, rather than their standard 16-18 hour assay, coleoptile elongation was much less sensitive to 2,4-D than to IAA or NAA - perhaps suggesting that the auxin receptor does have low intrinsic affinity for 2,4-D. It was also observed (Ray et al., 1977 a,b; Dohrmann et al., 1978) that analogue binding affinity was differentially regulated by supernatant factor (SF), a low molecular weight modifier of auxin binding whose removal is largely responsible for the improved NAA binding obtained by washing and repelleting membrane preparations. SF lowers the binding affinity for NAA without affecting site number (Fig. 5.3). On the other hand, in the presence of SF the overall biological activity-binding affinity correlation was somewhat improved, since the anomalous affinity of certain ligands with little or no auxin activity (e.g. PAA, phenylurea) was greatly reduced, while the binding affinity for some analogues, including 2,4-D was actually enhanced. It was therefore suggested that SF might function as a natural regulator of auxin activity. The regulation appeared to be mainly of site 1, conferring an affinity pattern closer to that of the more auxin-specific site 2 (Dohrmann et al., 1978).

SF was soon isolated and identified (Venis and Watson, 1978) as a mixture of 6-methoxy-2-benzoxazolinone (MBOA) and 6,7-dimethoxy-2-benzoxazolinone (DMBOA, Fig. 5.4). The parent compound 2-benzoxazolinone (BOA) was also found, but in much smaller amount. These are known natural products in maize and in certain other Gramineae, and have been implicated in resistance of cereals to fungi, insects and chloro-s-triazine herbicides (Klun et al., 1970 and references therein). In the intact plant the compounds occur as glucosides (I), from which the benzoxazinones (II) are released enzymically upon cell damage, e.g. by pathogenic attack or by homogenization. On warming

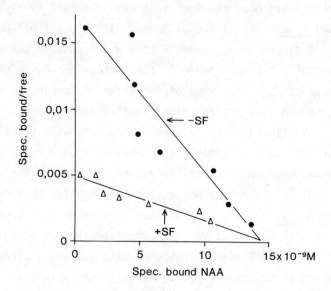

Fig. 5.3 - Effect of supernatant factor (SF) on saturable NAA-^{14}C
binding by maize membranes enriched in ER by sucrose gradient
centrifugation (Dohrmann et al., 1978)

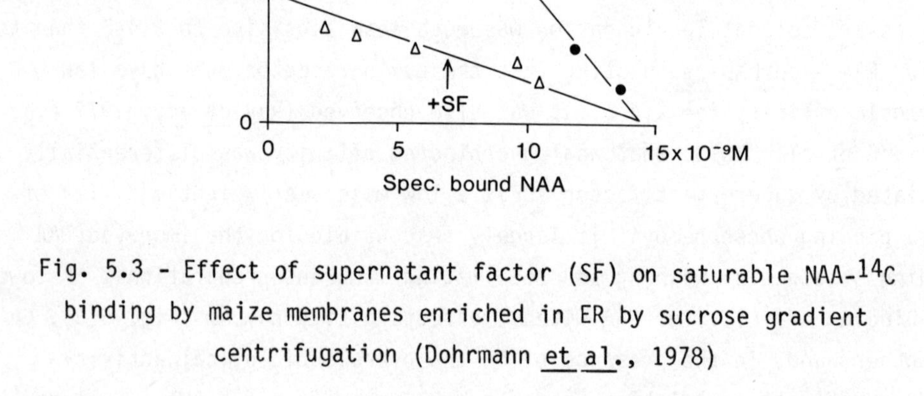

BOA : $R_1 = R_2 = H$
MBOA : $R_1 = OCH_3$, $R_2 = H$
DMBOA : $R_1 = R_2 = OCH_3$

Fig. 5.4 - Benzoxazolinones and precursors in maize

Table 5.2   Inhibitory effects of benzoxazolinones and benzoxazinones
(10 μg/ml) on NAA binding to maize coleoptile membranes and on
IAA-induced growth of oat coleoptiles (Venis, 1980)

Compound	% inhibition of binding	% inhibition of growth
DMBOA	69	78
DIBOA*	48	46
MBOA	36	44
HBOA*	14	29
5-Cl BOA	12	26
BOA	8	17

* HBOA and DIBOA are, respectively, 2-hydroxy-and 2,4-dihydroxy-1,4-
benzoxazin-3-one

in dilute aqueous solution the aglucones undergo ring contraction to produce
the benzoxazolinones III (Fig. 5.4). MBOA and DMBOA were isolated by
following inhibition of NAA-receptor binding during purification, a
convenient measure of SF activity. Both compounds are active in such assays
(Fig. 5.5), DMBOA being about 50 times more active than MBOA; BOA is only
weakly active. The compounds were also found to inhibit auxin-induced growth
of oat coleoptiles and the relative activity of BOA, MBOA, and DMBOA in such
assays correlated well with their inhibitory action on auxin-receptor
binding. This correlation was subsequently extended to other analogues
(Table 5.2). The benzoxazinone group of compounds has a very restricted
species distribution, occurring only in a few Gramineae (see references in
Venis and Watson, 1978). They cannot, therefore, have a general role in
auxin physiology, though it is not inconceivable that they do have a
regulatory function in the particular species concerned. Nevertheless, the
good correlation between the activity of the benzoxazolinones in inhibiting
on the one hand auxin-induced growth and on the other hand auxin-binding
site interaction is significant in providing evidence that these binding
sites may represent physiological receptor sites for auxin action.

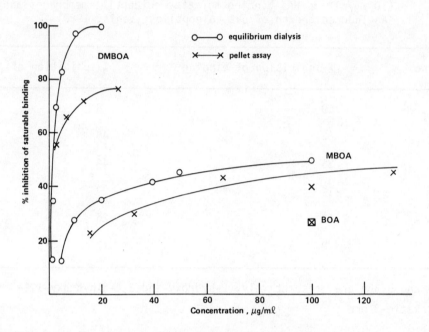

Fig. 5.5 - Benzoxazolinone inhibition of NAA binding to membrane-bound
(pellet assay) or solubilized (equilibrium dialysis; see 5.1.3)
receptors in maize (Venis and Watson, 1978)

5.1.2 Active-site modification

General group-modifying reagents and site-directed irreversible
inhibitors (affinity labels) have been used extensively in probing the
active sites of enzymes and of cholinergic and hormone receptors in animals.
The first compounds to be applied as potential auxin affinity labels (Venis,
1977b) were the diazonium salts of 2-chloro-4-aminophenoxyacetic acid (CAPA)
and of 2,5-dichloro-3-aminobenzoic acid (Chloramben) - Fig. 5.6. When maize
coleoptile membranes were treated at various pH values with these diazonium
salts, then pelleted from the reaction medium and resuspended at pH 5.5,
their ability to bind NAA-^{14}C was impaired in comparison with control
membranes incubated similarly but without diazonium salt. Diazo-CAPA was
effective only at pH 8-9, while inhibition by diazo-Chloramben was largely
independent of reaction pH over the range pH 6-9 (Fig. 5.7). Because
modification by diazo-Chloramben could be carried out at a pH close to the

optimum NAA-binding value, pH 5.5, it was possible to show that prior
addition of unlabelled NAA $(2.5 \times 10^{-5}M)$ to the membranes protected the
binding sites against inhibition by this diazonium analogue. This ligand
protection experiment suggested that the compound did indeed react at the

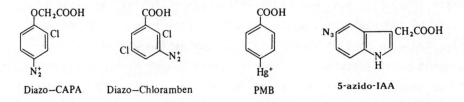

Diazo—CAPA   Diazo—Chloramben   PMB   5-azido-IAA

Fig. 5.6 - Site-directed inhibitors of auxin binding

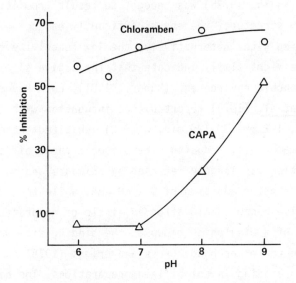

Fig. 5.7 - Effect of reaction pH on inhibition by diazonium salts of
CAPA or Chloramben (0.15 mM) of NAA-^{14}C binding by maize
coleoptile membranes (Venis, 1977b)

active auxin-binding site. From the different pH dependences of reaction, it
was proposed that diazo-Chloramben modified a histidine residue, while
diazo-CAPA reacted with tyrosine or lysine. Arguments based on the pH
profile of NAA binding also suggested the presence of a histidine (possibly

a second residue) at the binding site, and in addition an aspartate or glutamate residue. However, the latter suggestion derived from the charge separation theory's premise of a fractional positive charge on the auxin ring and, as discussed earlier, this has since been questioned by the studies of Farrimond et al. (1978, 1980, 1981).

Similar experiments with -SH reagents showed that 0.05-0.1 mM p-mercuri-benzoate (PMB, Fig. 5.6) was highly effective in inhibiting auxin-binding activity of the membranes, while the other thiol reagents tested were ineffective even at 1 mM (Venis, 1977b). Inhibition was reversed by subsequent brief addition of thiols (glutathione or dithiothreitol) and could be greatly reduced if NAA (10^{-5}M) was added before PMB. Comparable data were subsequently obtained by Cross and Briggs (1978) with solubilized membrane preparations. It was therefore suggested that PMB modified a cysteine residue at the active site. The effectiveness of PMB relative to other thiol reagents (Venis, 1977b) was thought to result from its general similarity to an auxin structure, thereby significantly enhancing its affinity for the binding site. Alternatively, the low reactivity of aliphatic -SH reagents might simply indicate that the active site cysteine residue is in a hydrophobic environment (Rubery, 1981). Both Ray et al. (1977a) and Dohrmann et al. (1978) reported that incubation with dithioerythritol (DTE, 1-2 mM, 90-120 min. at 0°C) inhibited subsequent auxin binding by the membranes, reducing site number without affecting affinity. This inhibition was largely reversed by oxidants and could be partly prevented by the prior addition of 0.1 mM NAA, while the physiologically inactive benzoic acid afforded little or no protection even at 1 mM. The presence of a disulphide group at the binding site was therefore inferred. On the other hand, Cross and Briggs (1978) found no effect of DTE on auxin binding in solubilized preparations. The basis for this discrepancy has not been clarified.

More recently the presence of an arginine residue at the auxin-binding site has been inferred from inactivation of membrane-NAA-^{3}H binding by phenylglyoxal (PGO); binding activity was protected by the inclusion of unlabelled NAA during the modification reaction (Nave and Benveniste, 1984). In the protection experiments, both the modification reaction and binding assay were carried out at pH 7.0, a compromise pH that is sub-optimal for PGO-arginine reaction and supra-optimal for auxin binding, necessitating rather high concentrations of PGO for inhibition (15 mM) and of NAA for protection (1 mM). If binding was performed under optimal conditions (pH 5.5, following a modification reaction at high pH), no PGO inhibition was observed and it was suggested (though without any other evidence) that the PGO-binding site adduct is unstable at the lower pH. Scatchard analysis of a pH 7.0 experiment (Fig. 5.8) indicated that PGO reduced site number

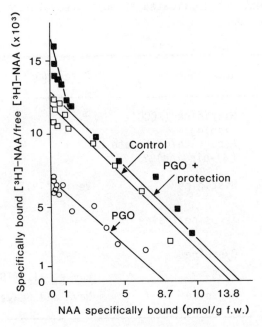

Fig. 5.8 - Scatchard analysis of NAA binding to maize membranes after incubation for 60 min at 30°C ±15mM PGO.
'Protection' = 1 mM NAA present during this incubation
(Navé and Benveniste, 1984)

without changing binding affinity for NAA ($K_d = 10^{-6}$M at pH 7.0). However, the reaction conditions used (60 min. at 30°C) can be expected to reduce binding activity markedly (Ray et al., 1977a) and the higher affinity sites (K_d ca. 2.5×10^{-7}M) apparent following NAA-protected PGO incubation (Fig. 5.8) may reflect partial preservation by the auxin of the intrinsic affinity of unincubated membrane sites. The latter data were not available for comparison, nor was an 'NAA-protected control' Scatchard plot, which presumably should show a set of higher affinity sites also.

Table 5.3 summarises the various suggestions that have been made concerning the possible amino acid environment of the active auxin-binding site.

Various azido-auxins have been explored as potential photoaffinity labels by Leonard and co-workers, the general strategy being to allow the compound to bind in the dark and then fix it _in situ_ by photolytic generation of the

Table 5.3   Amino-acid residues implicated at auxin receptor sites in maize membranes

Observation	Inference	Reference
1. pH Dependence of auxin binding	Histidine (-COO'-binding) Aspartate/glutamate (δ+-binding) ?	
2. Diazo-Chloramben inhibition at pH 6	Histidine	Venis (1977b)
3. Diazo-CAPA inhibition at pH 8-9	Tyrosine/lysine	
4. Inhibition by PMB	Cysteine	
5. Inhibition by DTE	-S-S- ?	Ray et al. (1977a)
6. Inhibition by PGO	Arginine	Navé and Benveniste (1984)

? indicates that these assignments have been questioned (see text)

highly reactive nitrene. The azido analogue of CAPA (i.e. 2-chloro-4-azido-phenoxyacetic acid) and a related azido derivative were first prepared (Leonard et al., 1975), but the 4-, 5-, and 6-azido IAA derivatives were subsequently found to have much better auxin activity (Melhado et al., 1981) and it is these compounds that have been investigated further. All the compounds compete for NAA-^{14}C binding by maize membranes in the dark, with affinities similar to that of IAA itself (Jones, A.M. et al., 1984a). Incubation with 5-azido IAA (Fig. 5.6) followed by UV irradiation led to a reduction in available NAA binding sites without affecting binding affinity. In addition, since NAA and IAA, but not benzoic acid or tryptophan, were able to protect against such site inactivation, it was considered that

5-azido IAA was reacting at or near the active site. The compound was then prepared tritiated to high specific activity and used to photo-label maize membrane preparations (Jones, A.M. et al., 1984b). The labelled membranes were extracted with 5M urea-1% Triton X-100 and the solubilized radioactive proteins were fractionated by various means. HPLC gel permeation (Fig. 5.9)

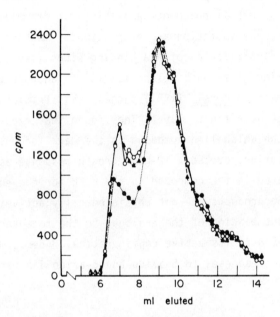

Fig. 5.9 - Radioactivity profiles of photolabeled maize membrane proteins on an Altex TSK-3000 column. Samples photolyzed with 2×10^{-6}M 5-azido-7-^{3}H-IAA alone (o), plus 10^{-4}M IAA (●) or plus 10^{-4}M NAA (▲) (Jones, A.M. et al., 1984b)

showed that radioactivity in the first peak, close to the void volume, was reduced if IAA was present during photolysis, whereas NAA had little or no protective effect. Gel isoelectric focussing and SDS gel electrophoresis also revealed selective reduction of labelling by IAA, but not by NAA. Because of the apparently low affinity of the labelled proteins for NAA and because the transport inhibitor TIBA (though not NPA) also afforded some protection against photo-labelling, it was suggested that the IAA-protected radioactive proteins were more likely to be concerned with auxin transport than with auxin perception. In this case, since 5-azido IAA does inactivate

83

NAA-binding sites of the site 1/2 type (Jones, A.M. et al., 1984a) the question arises as to why these proteins did not appear to be labelled. It was thought that the theoretical maximum labelling of such sites might be close to the detectable limit or, since the membrane solubilization procedure used removed only half of the radioactivity, that auxin-binding proteins might remain unextracted (Jones, A.M. et al., 1984b).

The photo-labelling obtained is clearly far from site-specific, but there should be scope for further improvement, possibly, for example, labelling in vivo, followed by membrane isolation and extraction by methods known to effect quantitative solubilization of NAA binding sites (Venis, 1977c, see next section). Labelling after such solubilization is another possibility. Results reported by Melhado et al. (1984) suggest that tritiated 4-azido IAA might be a more effective affinity label. They found that exposure of soybean sections to the unlabelled compound in the dark for only one hour, followed by UV irradiation, evoked a 12-hour growth response as great as that in tissue incubated in the compound in the dark for the entire 12-hour period. Since the photoproducts are not physiologically active, this result suggested that covalent binding of the analogue to the receptor site may have locked the receptor in its active configuration. Under similar conditions, the growth responses to 5-azido and 6-azido IAA were less pronounced.

5.1.3 Solubilization and purification

Auxin-binding activity in maize membranes can be readily solubilized by Triton X-100 (Batt et al., 1976; Ray et al., 1977a; Cross et al., 1978), but such extracts are not amenable to extensive purification. However, use of a modified acetone powder technique enabled the binding sites to be obtained in a buffer-soluble form without recourse to detergent treatment (Venis, 1977c) and kinetic analysis suggested the presence of two sets of binding sites in these extracts, with dissociation constants very similar to those reported for site 1 and site 2 in the membrane-bound state (see Table 5.1). The binding species appeared to be proteins and purification of about 100-fold was obtained by ion-exchange and gel permeation chromatography. Subsequent introduction of alternative and additional chromatographic steps on various liganded Sepharose columns (e.g. poly(U)-, heparin-, aminohexyl (AH)-Sepharose; Venis, 1980) led to still greater purification (Fig. 5.10,

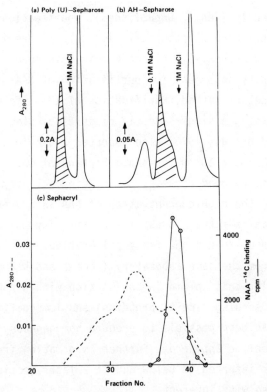

Fig. 5.10 - Purification of post-DEAE auxin-binding proteins from maize membranes. The shaded areas denote the auxin-binding fractions that were pooled and applied to the subsequent column (Venis, 1980)

Table 5.4   Purification of auxin-binding proteins from maize membranes (from 260 g of shoots. Venis, 1980)

Fraction	Total binding dpm	Total protein mg	Specific activity dpm/mg
Crude extract	559,747	194.50	2,878
DEAE Bio-Gel	303,398	8.21	36,943
Poly(U)-Sepharose	216,000	1.13	192,000
AH-Sepharose	141,704	0.54	262,416
Sephacryl	74,666	0.15	493,823 (mean) 564,553 (max)

Table 5.4). More recently (Venis, unpublished), modifications to the chromatographic buffers have substantially improved recoveries. Tappeser et al. (1981) have used 2-hydroxy-3,5-diiodobenzoic acid coupled to Epoxy-Sepharose as an affinity adsorbent for purification of NAA-binding proteins solubilized by the acetone method. Purification of 13-34-fold was obtained by salt elution, yielding a single kinetic class of binding sites, K_d ca. 2×10^{-7}M. (Cross and Briggs, 1978, also reported a single population of solubilized sites, $K_d = 5 \times 10^{-8}$M for NAA.) Elution of the affinity column with NAA (0.1 mM) also removed protein, but binding activity was not determined because of the high concentration of NAA in the eluate. The degree of purification is rather modest for an affinity column and the column required two hours/overnight for equilibration. However, a recent preliminary report from the same laboratory (Löbler and Klämbt, 1984) indicated that by using this column in conjunction with a control blocked spacer arm column (adsorbing 'inert' proteins) and immunoaffinity chromatography, it had been possible to prepare homogeneous auxin-binding protein and a monospecific antiserum. Further information from this preliminary report is referred to below and in a later section, and full publication is awaited with interest.

The apparent molecular weight of the solubilized binding proteins by gel permeation chromatography has been the subject of some debate. On Sephadex G100, Venis (1977c) obtained a possibly heterogeneous binding peak, in the 40,000-47,000 daltons range. Cross et al. (1978) reported a molecular weight of 90,000 for the auxin-binding sites from Triton-extracted membranes, but this appears to correspond to the size of a detergent-protein micelle. Subsequently, however, Cross and Briggs (1978) observed a similar size auxin-binding peak (80,000 daltons) by both detergent and acetone powder methods, and Cross et al. (1978) suggested that failure to include a protease inhibitor, such as PMSF (phenylmethylsulphonylfluoride), in the initial membrane homogenization buffer could have caused receptor degradation to the size previously reported in acetone powder extracts (Venis, 1977b). Cross and Briggs (1978) used a different gel permeation column (Bio-Gel A 1.5 m), run at higher pH and ionic strength, claiming aggregation to 200,000 daltons in the absence of 0.1 M NaCl. Attempts were made to resolve the molecular weight discrepancy, using a variety of extraction and gel filtration conditions (Venis, 1980). However, irrespective of ionic strength, gel type, or the use of PMSF, only molecular weights in the 40,000-44,000 range were observed (Table 5.5). Subsequently Murphy (1980a) and Tappeser et al. (1981), both using PMSF, have obtained molecular weights on Sephadex G100 of 43,700 and 45,000 respectively for maize membrane proteins solubilized by the acetone method. The report of Cross and Briggs (1978) therefore stands alone and it seems likely that for some reason, possibly a varietal peculiarity, their binding protein extracts were subject to aggregation.

Table 5.5   Elution of auxin-binding activity by gel filtration of crude maize membrane acetone powder extracts under different conditions (Venis, 1980)

PMSF in extraction medium	Gel permeation conditions			Apparent M.W. at binding peak
	Column	Buffer	NaCl	
a.None	Sephadex G100	10 mM citrate-acetate, pH 5.5	0	43,800
b.0.25 mM	Sephadex G100	10 mM citrate-acetate, pH 5.5	0	43,800
c.0.25 mM	Sephadex G75	10 mM citrate-acetate, pH 5.5	0	39,300
d.0.25 mM	Sephadex G75	10 mM tris-HCl, pH 7.6	0.1 M	42,000
e.0.25 mM	Bio-Gel A 0.5 m	10 mM tris-HCl, pH 7.6	0.1 M	40,700
f.0.25 mM	Bio-Gel A 1.5 m	10 mM tris-HCl, pH 7.6	0.1 M	41,000
g.0.25 mM	Bio-Gel A 1.5 m	10 mM tris-HCl, pH 7.6	0	40,800

Other questions not yet properly resolved are the number of protein sub-units and whether there is more than one discrete binding protein species. Venis (1980) was able to resolve two binding peaks either by Sephadex G15 isoelectric focussing (IEF) of post-DEAE fractions, or by shallow salt gradient elution of crude extracts on DEAE Bio-Gel. However, IEF over the pH range required for resolution (pH 3.5-5) gave only 10-15% recovery of activity and the resolved DEAE column peaks were not purified further.

Fractions purified according to the schedule in Table 5.4 showed two predominant bands on both non-dissociating and sodium dodecyl sulphate (SDS) gel electrophoresis (Venis, 1980). The main SDS gel bands were at 40,000 and 46,000 daltons, agreeing with gel filtration estimates and suggesting that the proteins are monomeric. It was not possible to establish that these represent two binding proteins, since no activity could be recovered by elution from non-dissociating gels. The most purified fractions of Tappeser et al. (1981) - from gel filtration after affinity chromatography - showed several faint bands on SDS gels, at 45, 35, 33, 26, 25, 20 and 19 kilo-daltons, and it was suggested that the binding protein(s) are dimeric. The preliminary report of Löbler and Klämbt (1984) indicated that only one band, at 20,000 daltons, was visible on SDS gels after immunoaffinity purification. Further information is needed to evaluate this claim, but availability of antibodies could certainly help to resolve several areas of uncertainty.

5.1.4 Physiological relevance

So far this Chapter has dealt with the general kinetics, distribution and chemical properties of auxin-binding sites in maize membranes, but only briefly with physiological significance. The binding proteins do not appear to be involved in auxin metabolism, insofar as they can be resolved from IAA oxidase activity and have no detectable auxin conjugating activity (Venis, 1980). In both detergent-treated and acetone-treated membrane extracts, binding activity can also be separated from ATPase (Cross et al., 1978; Venis, 1980). Apart from having appropriate binding affinities and selectivity between auxin analogues that is generally consistent with relative physiological activities, support for a receptor function for these and related binding sites has come from several pieces of correlative evidence:

1. The first of these has already been discussed, namely the correlation between effects of benzoxazolinones on auxin-binding site interaction and on auxin-induced growth (Fig. 5.5; Table 5.2).

2. Maize mesocotyl membranes also bind NAA (Ray et al., 1977b) and the binding proteins appear to be similar to those of coleoptiles in molecular size and ion-exchange behaviour (Venis, unpublished results). Walton and Ray (1981) found that auxin binding and auxin-induced elongation decreased in

parallel down the length of the mesocotyl (Fig. 5.11). Furthermore, exposure to red light reduced auxin responsiveness and auxin binding activity of mesocotyls (but not coleoptiles) with a similar time course and to a similar extent (Fig. 5.12). Reduced NAA binding was brought about by a decrease in site number without influencing binding affinity (K_d 2 x 10^{-7}M) and this effect corresponded to the way in which red light inhibited growth, which

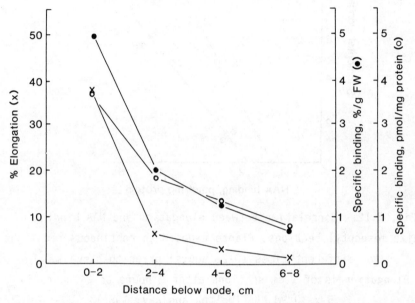

Fig. 5.11 - Auxin-stimulated elongation and NAA binding as a function of position along the maize mesocotyl (Walton and Ray, 1981)

was to reduce the maximum response to NAA without affecting the NAA concentration at which the half-maximal response was obtained (ca. 2 x 10^{-7}M). Earlier, Normand et al. (1977) had failed to observe any effect of red light (10 min.) on auxin binding by maize membranes from either coleoptiles or mesocotyls, but they appear to have homogenized the tissue immediately after irradiation, whereas Walton and Ray (1981) found that at least four hours between onset of seedling irradiation and harvest was needed for any significant reduction in binding.

3. Comparing maize coleoptiles of different ages (sizes), it was found that as coleoptile size increased, auxin binding and auxin responsiveness (measured as maximum growth increment) were reduced in concert (Kearns, 1982).

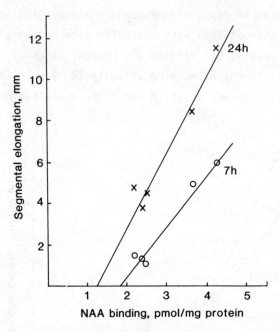

Fig. 5.12 - Correlation between elongation and NAA binding of
maize mesocotyl sections. Plants exposed to continuous red light
for different times (0-28 hours) prior to harvest.
Elongation is of 1 cm sections after 7 hours or 24 hours in
$5 \times 10^{-6}M$ NAA (Walton and Ray, 1981)

4. Apical 1 cm sections of oat coleoptiles are far more auxin-sensitive
and show higher auxin binding than basal sections (Fig. 5.13; data from
Kearns, 1982).

5. In maize coleoptiles the reverse situation was found, i.e. basal
sections, somewhat surprisingly, were more auxin-responsive than apical
sections, but they also had greater auxin binding activity (Kearns, 1982).

The above evidence is all circumstantial, but taken overall is fairly
persuasive. The fact that auxin sensitivity and auxin binding remain
correlated as described in oat and in maize is particularly suggestive. In
addition, there are now two more direct pieces of evidence pointing to a
receptor role for these membrane binding sites. Firstly, maize auxin-binding
proteins solubilized from the membranes and partly purified on a DEAE column

(at which stage the protein fraction still contains ATPase activity) have been incorporated by aqueous diffusion into a synthetic bilayer lipid membrane, across which a fixed potential was applied (Thompson, M. *et al.*, 1983). Addition of NAA followed by ATP produced an immediate rise in transmembrane current (Fig. 5.14). All three components (protein, auxin, ATP) were required for the response to occur, but the order of addition was

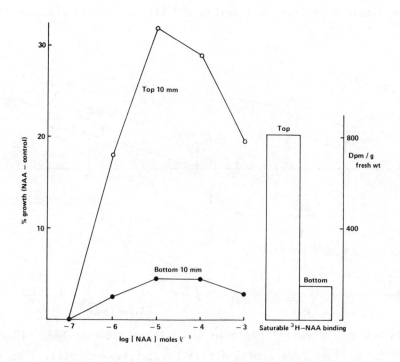

Fig. 5.13 - Comparison of NAA-induced elongation (6 hours) and NAA-^{3}H binding in top and bottom 10 mm sections of oat coleoptiles (Kearns, 1982)

not critical. No response occurred with the physiologically inactive benzoic acid, but subsequent addition of NAA elicited the electrochemical response (Fig. 5.14). The pH dependence of the response, together with the known pH dependence of auxin binding, was consistent with the operation of a proton-translocating ATPase, stimulated by auxin plus receptor. This reconstitution experiment thus provides direct support for the proton pump hypothesis of auxin action, and represents the first biochemical response to be associated with a hormone-binding protein in plants. It is hoped that future work along these lines will permit a more detailed examination of factors such as auxin and nucleotide specificity.

The other piece of direct evidence has, at the time of writing, appeared only as a preliminary report at the 1984 FEBS Congress (Löbler and Klämbt, 1984). A monospecific antiserum directed against maize membrane auxin-binding proteins and prepared via affinity and immunoaffinity chromatography, as outlined earlier, was tested for its ability to block an auxin-

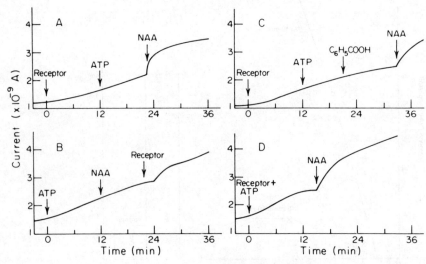

Fig. 5.14 - Electrochemical response of auxin receptor to NAA, ATP and C_6H_5COOH for various orders of addition to positive-potential side of membrane (A, B and C). Response for transmembrane addition of receptor/ATP and NAA (D). Final concentrations: receptor $6 \times 10^{-9}M$, ATP $4 \times 10^{-6}M$, NAA and C_6H_5COOH $2 \times 10^{-5}M$. (Thompson et al., 1983)

induced growth response. The response examined, inrolling of split maize coleoptiles, was inhibited if the tissue was incubated in the antiserum for six hours prior to auxin addition, whereas pre-incubation in non-immune serum was without effect. Details of this work await publication, but ostensibly these results point to two important conclusions. Firstly, they reinforce the suggestion that these binding sites are auxin receptors.

Secondly, since it is improbable that the antiserum was able to enter undamaged cells, auxin receptors involved in cell expansion must be located at the outer face of the plasma membrane. This is not to say that similar or identical receptors, perhaps mediating other auxin responses, do not also occur intracellularly. Immunohistochemical examination suggested that the binding sites were largely restricted to the outer epidermal cells. When full experimental details appear, it will be important to ascertain that the antiserum is truly monospecific for the auxin-binding protein(s). If so, it will be of considerable interest to see, inter alia, whether immuno-chemically-related proteins occur in other species, whether auxin-dependent growth responses can be blocked in these species, and indeed whether auxin-induced responses other than growth can be inhibited by antiserum.

5.2. SITE III AND AUXIN TRANSPORT: MAIZE AND ZUCCHINI MEMBRANES

At the beginning of this Chapter it was noted that Dohrmann et al. (1978) had obtained indications of a third auxin-binding site in maize membranes, site III, that was characterized by a higher binding affinity for 2,4-D than for NAA. This binding was studied further by Jacobs and Hertel (1978), principally in zucchini hypocotyl membranes, where it was more readily detectable and where site I binding (PAA-saturable) was minimal. Binding of IAA-^{14}C in zucchini membranes was relatively insensitive to displacement by NAA and was stimulated by the transport inhibitors TIBA and NPA (e.g. 10^{-5}M TIBA nearly doubled saturable binding). Differential centrifugation and isopycnic centrifugation on sucrose and metrizamide gradients suggested that the IAA-binding activity was associated with plasma membrane fractions. There was an approximate correlation between relative activities of analogues as auxin transport inhibitors and as competitors of auxin binding (Table 5.6), the major anomalies being NAA, which strongly inhibits IAA transport but competes very poorly for binding, and the isomeric 2-NAA which binds with much greater affinity than would be expected from its activity as a transport inhibitor. From this correlation, from the apparent plasma membrane localization, and from the effects of NPA and TIBA on binding, it was suggested that site III may represent an auxin transport site.

Table 5.6 Activities of auxins and analogues as inhibitors of auxin
transport and as competitors of IAA binding in zucchini.
C_{50} = concentration giving 50% inhibition of polar auxin
transport. K_d (apparent) = concentration giving 50% reduction
in saturable IAA-^{14}C binding (from Jacobs and Hertel, 1978)

Compound	Transport inhibition, C_{50} x 10^{-6}M	Binding competition, K_d x 10^{-6}M
NAA	2.5	79
(+) 2,4-DP	5.0	3.2
(-) 2,4-DP	10	50
2-NAA	32	0.5
NOA	100	3.2
IAA	100	1.6
2,4-D	320	5.0
4-CPIB*	320	200
PAA	1000	160
BA*	1000	2000

* 4-CPIB = 4-chlorophenoxyisobutyric acid. BA = benzoic acid

Although Jacobs and Hertel (1978) considered it highly unlikely that this
binding consisted of saturable transport into sealed vesicles, subsequent
investigation (Hertel et al., 1983) showed that 'site III binding' could in
fact be interpreted in just such terms, with uptake being drive by a proton
gradient and the whole system presenting an in vitro simulation of the
mechanism of auxin transport. The chemiosmotic model of auxin transport
(Rubery and Sheldrake, 1974) proposed that auxin moves across the plasma
membrane into the cytoplasm down a proton gradient (cell wall more acidic)
via a proton/auxin anion symport, Fig. 5.15. (In the cell-free system the
proton gradient derives from the pH difference between media of vesicle
preparation and of final resuspension.) Polarity of transport is achieved by
efflux of auxin through specific anion efflux carriers that are located in
the plasma membrane preferentially at the basal ends of transporting cells
(Fig. 5.15). Inhibitors of auxin transport are thought to block the auxin
efflux carrier (Sussman and Goldsmith, 1981). Thus, if 'site III binding'

represents net auxin uptake into sealed right side out plasmalemma vesicles, i.e. the net component of symport entry and anion efflux, then binding should be sensitive to protonophores that collapse the proton gradient, and should be stimulated by transport inhibitors such as NPA or TIBA. These are precisely the features of IAA binding that have been found in zucchini and

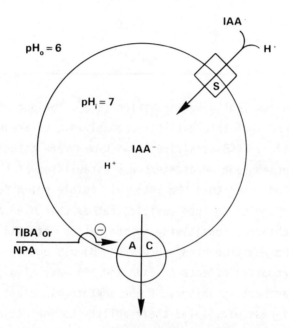

Fig. 5.15 - Hypothetical scheme of an outside-out plasma membrane vesicle or of a cell. S = specific, saturable auxin-H^+ symport: AC = specific, saturable auxin-anion-carrier which is non-competitively inhibited by TIBA and NPA. Driving force for the IAA-flux is provided by an H^+ gradient across the membrane (Hertel et al., 1983)

are illustrated in Table 5.7. The 'binding' is saturable by unlabelled IAA and is enhanced by TIBA, as found earlier by Jacobs and Hertel (1978). In addition, however, the proton ionophore FCCP (carbonyl cyanide 4-trifluoro-methoxyphenyl hydrazone) greatly reduces saturable IAA-^{14}C association, including the stimulated value in the presence of TIBA. Nigericin (a H^+/K^+ ionophore) was found to exert a similar effect. Jacobs and Hertel (1978) had

Table 5.7 Effect of FCCP and TIBA on IAA-^{14}C (10^{-7}M) association to
zucchini membranes prepared at pH 7.9 and assayed at pH 6.0
(from Hertel et al., 1983)

Added in assay	Membrane pellet cpm	
	Control	+FCCP
—	1046	728
TIBA, 3 x 10^{-6}M	1363	770
IAA, 3 x 10^{-5}M	590	520

noted that binding was labile to incubation at 0°C for one hour and Hertel
et al. (1983) showed that this was most probably due to breakdown of the pH
gradient. In addition, FCCP-sensitive IAA-^{14}C-membrane association was only
observed if a transmembrane pH gradient was established at the outset by
resuspension at a pH lower than the internal vesicle pH. A further
indication that accumulation into vesicles rather than binding was being
measured was the observed sensitivity to sonication, osmotic shock and
freeze-thawing, whereas true binding (of NPA-^{3}H) was unaffected by these
treatments. The promotive effects of TIBA and NPA were also observed with a
range of auxin transport inhibitors of the phytotropin class (see Chapter
4), whose effectiveness paralleled their ability to inhibit auxin transport.
Thus PBA, 2-(1-pyrenoyl) benzoic acid, the most potent transport inhibitor
known, was more effective than NPA, while the physiologically inactive
analogue 2-benzoylbenzoic acid (BBA) was also completely without effect on
in vitro IAA accumulation (Fig. 5.16).

Hertel (1983) proposed that the non-electrogenic uptake scheme depicted
in Fig. 5.15 should be amended to an electrogenic cotransport of IAA' with
two protons. This suggestion was based partly on approximate calculations
indicating that IAA accumulation was greater than the imposed proton
gradient, and partly on the observed stimulation of IAA uptake by the K^{+}
ionophore valinomycin when vesicles were pre-loaded with 20 mM K^{+} and
resuspended in low K^{+} medium (Table 5.8). Under these conditions valinomycin
can be expected to create a strong internal negative potential. When

potential generation was prevented by equimolar K^+ externally, valinomycin had no effect (Table 5.8), supporting the proposed electrogenic transport mechanism.

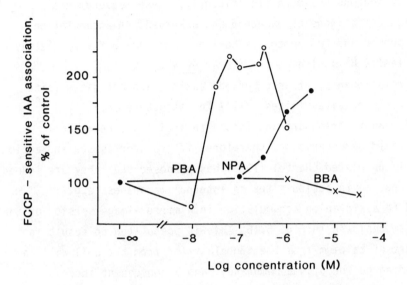

Fig. 5.16 - Effects of active (NPA, PBA) and inactive (BBA) phytotropins on FCCP-sensitive IAA-^{14}C accumulation by zucchini membrane vesicles (from Hertel et al., 1983)

Table 5.8 Effects of valinomycin and KCl on IAA-^{14}C association with zucchini hypocotyl membranes. Extraction medium contained 20 mM KCl. Reagent concentrations in resuspension media were 3×10^{-7}M (PBA) or 3×10^{-6}M (valinomycin = Val, and FCCP). From Hertel, 1983

Added in assay	IAA-^{14}C in pellet, cpm		
	Control	Valinomycin	Valinomycin + 20 mM Kcl
Control	698	1261	674
PBA	950	1830	967
PBA + FCCP	301	310	273

Further confirmation of this mechanism came from application of esr spectroscopic methods with spin-labelled nitroxide probes to measure the internal pH and volume of zucchini vesicles (Lomax and Melhorn, 1985). These showed that the vesicles were osmotically responsive (and therefore sealed) and did maintain an imposed pH gradient that slowly decayed with time and was dissipated by ionophores. More significantly, these measurements permitted precise comparisons of expected and observed IAA accumulation ratios for one proton and two proton mechanisms, and came out very clearly in favour of 1 IAA':2 H^+ stoichiometry (Lomax et al., 1985).

What is the relationship, if any, between auxin transport sites (site III) and auxin receptor sites (sites I/II)? The structure-activity relationships for auxin transport and for auxin action are remarkably similar and it would be surprising, therefore, if transport sites and action sites were wholly unrelated. Hertel (1983) has proposed that they are indeed homologous and that auxin action sites on internal membranes (e.g. tonoplast) lead to auxin anion accumulation in a mirror-image version of the sort of mechanism depicted in Fig. 5.15. This is postulated to result in counter-transport of calcium from the tonoplast (or from the cell wall in the case of binding to the plasma membrane), and a consequent increase in cytoplasmic calcium concentration, which triggers auxin action. Experimental evidence of IAA-calcium counterflow in polar auxin transport that is in general agreement with this model has been obtained (Guzman and de la Fuente, 1984). The tonoplastic calcium flow and hence the proposed tonoplast (and perhaps ER) auxin sites are regarded as the more important elements for auxin action, though this suggestion is not, of course, compatible with the preliminary data of Löbler and Klämbt (1984) suggesting that auxin action sites are located at the cell surface (see section 5.1.4). There is certainly considerable current interest in the possible role of calcium as a second messenger of plant hormone action and regulation by the calcium-calmodulin system, though the evidence to date is largely indirect (see Chapter 3).

5.3. MEMBRANE-BOUND SITES IN OTHER SPECIES

As noted earlier (5.1.4), oat coleoptile membranes also have auxin-binding activity, as do coleoptiles of wheat and rye (Kearns, 1982; Firn and Kearns, 1982). The characteristics of IAA-^{14}C binding to wheat coleoptile

membranes have recently been studied in greater detail by Zazimalova and
Kutacek (1985a), with promising results. One class of binding sites was
found, with a pH optimum (pH 5.2) and site concentration (60 pmol/g tissue)
similar to values observed in maize, but with a much higher affinity for IAA
(K_d 2 x 10^{-8}M). Interestingly, binding was found to be temperature-dependent
(Fig. 5.17), a 10 min. incubation at 20°C being optimal. Kearns (1982) had
measured binding (of NAA) at 0-5°C, the standard conditions used
for maize, but in wheat, binding at these low temperatures appears to be
only a small fraction of that observed at 20°C (Fig. 5.17). Binding
specificity was examined by measuring the ability of analogues to displace
IAA-^{14}C from the binding sites (Table 5.9). While there is an apparent
discrepancy between the IAA K_d determined by Scatchard analysis (2 x 10^{-8}M)
and that derived by correction (Cheng and Prusoff, 1973) from the C_{50} value
(10^{-7}M), there is nevertheless a remarkable correlation between binding
affinity and biological activity. In particular, the affinities of 2-NAA and
of IAA correspond better to their relative activities than in maize. Further

Table 5.9 Displacement of IAA-^{14}C (7.9 x 10^{-8}M) from wheat membrane binding
sites and comparison with auxin activity (from Zazimalova and
Kutacek, 1985a)

Compound	C_{50}, x 10^{-6}M	C^{*}_{50}	Relative auxin activity[1]
IAA	0.50	1.00	1.0
1-NAA	0.45	1.10	1.2
2-NAA	62	0.008	0.01
5-F-IAA	1.9	0.26	0.2
5-Cl-IAA	0.14	3.57	3.3
5-Br-IAA	1.9	0.26	0.3

C_{50} = concentration giving 50% displacement of saturable IAA-^{14}C binding
C^{*}_{50} = ratio IAA C_{50}:compound C_{50}
[1] wheat coleoptile straight growth test

data have been reported with a wider range of halogenated and dihalogenated IAAs (Zazimalova and Kutacek, 1985b). The excellent correlation was maintained and the results were considered broadly to conform to expectations from the auxin receptor map of Katekar (1979). It is to be hoped that this work can be confirmed and extended so that, for example, the relationship of these sites to those in maize can be evaluated. Quantitatively, the binding observed in wheat at 20°C (Fig. 5.17) is if anything greater than that seen in maize at lower temperatures, so the system should be readily amenable to further experimentation.

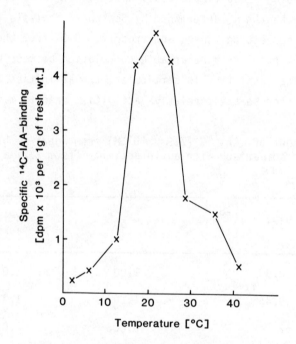

Fig. 5.17 - Effect of temperature on IAA binding to wheat membranes
(Zazimalova and Kutacek, 1985a)

Bhattacharyya and Biswas (1982) reported that a high affinity membranous IAA-binding site (K_d 6.8 x 10^{-7}M) was induced in wheat roots by one hour pretreatment in IAA (5 x 10^{-5}M), adding to the lower affinity site (K_d 7 x 10^{-6}M) already present in control roots. Induction of the higher affinity site was stated to be blocked by cycloheximide. Control coleoptile membranes contained two classes of binding site (K_d 2 x 10^{-7}M and 7 x 10^{-6}M) and, based partly on gel autoradiographs of pulse-labelled protein, it was suggested that the higher affinity site corresponded to the one induced in roots. Only sketches of gels were shown, however. These experiments were carried out with a 1000-12,000 g particulate fraction, whereas much 'lighter' fractions (e.g. 5000-50,000 g) are normally used in this type of work. It is worth noting that in some tissues saturable auxin 'binding' to heavy particulate fractions (10,000 g) has turned out to be resistant to protease and/or heat treatment (Kearns, 1982; Firn and Kearns, 1982). This information was not given for the oat sites, nor was it included in the report by Moloney and Pilet (1981) of NAA binding to 10,000 g fractions from maize roots (which was quantitatively much greater than to lighter fractions).

Another possible example of auxin regulation of its own binding site synthesis (perhaps comparable to similar such regulation by animal steroids) is the report by Trewavas (1980) of the appearance of IAA-binding sites (K_d ca. 10^{-6}M) in membrane preparations from artichoke tuber slices cultured in 10^{-6}M 2,4-D for 24 hours. Quantitatively, the level of saturable binding obtained was rather low, and the supply of sterile tissue was a further limitation to detailed investigation. Other tissues in which binding of IAA to particulate fractions has been reported are buds of light-grown peas (Jablonovic and Nooden, 1974), mung bean hypocotyls (Kasamo and Yamaki, 1976) and soybean hypocotyls (Williamson et al., 1977). In all cases saturable binding was only a small fraction of total binding, no kinetic data were presented and there was little or no information on binding specificity.

Pea tissues were also used by Döllstädt et al. (1976) who described saturable binding of IAA and certain substituted phenoxyacetic acids to particulate preparations from etiolated pea epicotyls and roots. Again, binding activities were rather low, but dissociation constants for IAA and MCPA were tentatively estimated at 10^{-6}M or lower, with 5 x 10^4 IAA- binding sites per cell. Displacement of IAA-^{14}C or MCPA-^{14}C from the binding sites by various phenoxyacetic acids was in general agreement with their relative auxin activities. Phenoxyacetic acids could displace IAA-^{14}C, but IAA did not compete for binding of labelled 4-chlorophenoxyacetic acid or MCPA and it was suggested that phenoxyacetic acids may bind to a site on the receptor that is distinct from the auxin-binding site and affect IAA binding allosterically. The possibility of distinct binding sites for phenoxyacetic acids could be of interest in relation to the herbicidal activity of these compounds. More recently, an abstract from Slone and Bilderback (1983) reported saturable, high affinity IAA binding to pea epicotyl membranes, with optimum binding at pH 4. However, from an ensuing abstract (Slone and Bilderback, 1984) it transpires that this 'binding' is in fact of the type described in the preceding section, i.e. it requires a pH gradient, is abolished by protonophores and appears to represent uptake into sealed vesicles. However, TIBA does not apparently increase the uptake of IAA (Bilderback, personal communication), though it would be of interest to know the effect of NPA on net uptake, given the clear demonstration of NPA binding sites (putative auxin efflux sites) in the same tissue (Jacobs and Gilbert, 1983).

Binding of NAA-^{14}C at a strongly acidic pH optimum (pH 4) has also been reported in fruit membranes of cucumber and strawberry (Narayanan et al., 1981 a,b). In cucumber a curvilinear Scatchard plot was obtained, but even using the steep part of the curve the apparent binding affinity was fairly low (1-2 x 10^{-5}M) and the site concentration high (1250 pmol/g tissue). With strawberry membranes, a linear Scatchard plot was obtained and somewhat higher NAA binding affinity (1.1 x 10^{-6}M, 100 pmol binding sites/g tissue). A good correlation was observed between competitive activity of auxin analogues and their ability to promote receptacle expansion. Bearing in mind that at the low pH used for binding in these studies a considerable transmembrane pH gradient could exist if the membranes were isolated as sealed vesicles, then there is the possibility that uptake rather than binding was being studied, as in peas. It would be of interest to see if the binding survives detergent or protonophore treatment.

Finally in this section we come to a rather better-characterized system, the auxin-binding sites of tobacco tissues, which have been studied by Libbenga and co-workers at Leiden - both soluble binding sites (discussed in the next section) and membrane-bound. The latter were first reported in cultured pith callus (Vreugdenhil et al., 1979), where they were found to

have many properties similar to those of the maize binding sites - pH
optimum (pH 5.0), sensitivity to heat and pronase treatment, binding
affinity for NAA-^{14}C (K_d 3 x 10^{-7}M) and site concentration (87 pmol/g). In
freshly-excised pith there were fewer binding sites (28 pmol/g). Specificity
was examined by analogue displacement of NAA-^{14}C. The apparent binding
affinities were approximately correlated with auxin activity, anomalies
being the low affinities for IAA (K_d 1.7 x 10^{-5}M) and TIBA (6.7 x 10^{-5}M). On
the other hand, the affinity for 2,4-D (K_d 3 x 10^{-6}M) was greater than in
maize (K_d 0.1 mM; Ray et al., 1977b) and more in keeping with the
physiological activity of this compound. It was not possible to establish
membrane localization by gradient centrifugation, nor could the binding
sites be solubilized either by detergent treatment or by the acetone method
used in maize. A further, more major departure from the characteristics of
the maize sites was the time- and temperature-dependence of binding, the
optimum incubation conditions being 36°C for 30 min. (Fig. 5.18). This
behaviour subsequently enabled the non-equilibrium binding kinetics to be
determined using a glass fibre filtration method (Maan et al., 1983). These
studies were more conveniently carried out at 25°C, since at the lower
temperature the rate of loading was somewhat lower (1-2 hours to binding
maximum), but the binding was then stable for several hours (note binding
reduction beyond 30 min. in Fig. 5.18). At equilibrium, centrifugation and

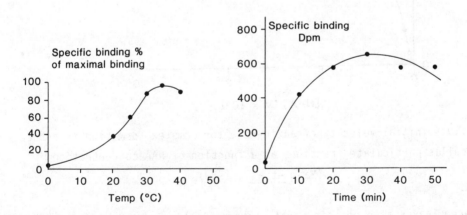

Fig. 5.18 - Temperature-dependence (left) and time-dependence (right)
of saturable NAA-^{14}C binding by particulate preparations from tobacco
callus (Vreugdenhil et al., 1979)

filtration assays yielded comparable K_d values for NAA at 25^0C of ca. 2 x 10^{-7}M. The rate of dissociation of the NAA-binding site complex was not a straightforward linear function, indicating that at least two binding complexes are involved. Measurement of the initial rate of site loading (V_0) as a function of NAA concentration (Fig. 5.19) confirmed that binding was more complex than a one-to-one hormone-receptor interaction. Moreover, the biphasic saturation curve of Fig. 5.19 suggested that the different binding events are not independent but are coupled in some way. A co-operative binding system involving four hormone molecules and one receptor molecule was proposed that fitted the kinetic observations, though it was recognized that other models could not be excluded.

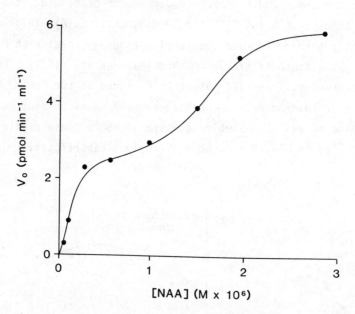

Fig. 5.19 - Initial velocity of auxin-receptor complex formation in tobacco callus particulate fractions as a function of NAA concentration
(Maan et al., 1983)

Tobacco leaves also contain particulate auxin-binding sites (Vreugdenhil et al., 1980). Protoplasts freshly isolated from such leaves did not bind NAA-^{14}C, but acquired binding activity after 3-4 days in culture, coincident with the first cell divisions, and attained maximum activity after 10 days. The affinity for NAA was similar in protoplasts and leaves $(4\text{-}5 \times 10^{-7}\text{M})$. There was evidence to suggest that the binding sites were destroyed by proteolytic contaminants in the digestion enzymes used for protoplast isolation, indicating that the sites may be located in the exterior face of the plasma membrane. If so, the system could offer interesting possibilities for studies on biosynthesis and function.

In batch-cultured tobacco cells, auxin binding was apparently modulated during the growth cycle (Vreugdenhil _et al._, 1981). The K_d for NAA (_ca._ $2 \times 10^{-7}\text{M}$) did not change appreciably, but the binding site concentration did. After subculture, the number of binding sites, following an initial decline, increased more rapidly than membrane protein or cell number (Fig. 5.20), so that the site number per cell increased 4-fold between day 1 and day 6. The functional significance of this increase is not clear; it was

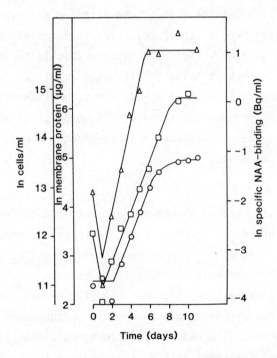

Fig. 5.20.- Semi-logarithmic plots of the growth of tobacco cells in batch culture measured by cell number (o), membrane protein (□) and saturable NAA-^{14}C binding (Δ) (Vreugdenhil _et al._, 1981)

suggested that the increase might be needed for cell expansion at the end of the division phase. A further example of binding site modulation comes in a recent report from Maan et al. (1985b) that in both suspension cultures and callus cultures, auxin-membrane binding disappears if 2,4-D replaces NAA plus kinetin in the culture medium. Since the cell doubling times in the two media were comparable, this suggests that the binding sites are not connected with cell division. There did, however, seem to be a possible connection with rooting ability, since calli on solid media with 2,4-D were unable to generate roots, whereas those on NAA plus kinetin did produce roots. It was considered that the low affinity of the tobacco binding sites for IAA (K_d 1.7 x 10^{-5}M) was compatible with the high IAA concentration needed for root induction.

5.4 SOLUBLE BINDING SITES

The first attempt to examine binding of a plant hormone to soluble protein was by Siegel and Galston (1953), who detected Salkowski-positive material in precipitates from trichloracetic acid-treated mixtures of pea root protein and IAA. Currently there is only one soluble auxin-binding system - from tobacco - that is being investigated at all systematically, and this will be discussed in section 5.4.2. First, mention will be made of a system from coconuts that was the subject of several publications in the 1970s, and finally a number of isolated reports, mostly considered artefactual, will be discussed.

5.4.1 Coconuts

In a series of papers, Biswas and co-workers outlined the properties of a putative auxin receptor, n-IRP (nucleoplasmic IAA receptor protein), prepared from nuclei of immature coconut endosperm (Mondal et al., 1972; Biswas et al., 1975; Roy and Biswas, 1977). In a homologous RNA synthesising system, activity was doubled by n-IRP, when IAA (10^{-5}M) was also present. Most of the enhanced RNA synthesis was the result of increased chain initiation, while hybridization and gel electrophoretic analysis of reaction products suggested that new kinds of RNA were produced in the stimulated reaction. n-IRP was reported to be a single polypeptide of 100,000 daltons and to bind to DNA-^{3}H. Binding was further enhanced by IAA, at an optimum concentration of 10^{-7}M. Equilibrium dialysis data (at one ligand concentration only) suggested that n-IRP binds IAA and 2,4-D, but not the inactive compound benzoic acid. From a fuller analysis of IAA binding, the K_d was estimated at 7.5×10^{-6}M.

An IAA-lysine affinity column (Venis, 1971) was used to purify n-IRP, eluted with 1M KSCN (Roy and Biswas, 1977). In addition, the same paper reported the similar affinity purification of another auxin receptor c-IRP (chromosomal IAA receptor protein), obtained from the chromatin fraction. Binding was assayed by a dextran-charcoal method, and Scatchard analysis indicated two sets of IAA-binding sites, with K_d values of 5.8×10^{-8}M and 8.15×10^{-6}M. The latter was described as non-specific binding, though the dissociation constant is in fact very similar to that given for n-IRP. The molecular weight was reported to be 70,000 daltons by SDS gel electrophoresis. The description of c-IRP isolation stated that the crude material was passed through CM-cellulose (which would remove any n-IRP present; Mondal et al., 1972) prior to affinity chromatography. However, the legend to the affinity column profile indicated that the total non-histone protein fraction obtained after chromatin solubilization and re-association was used. Since it is also unclear as to whether the Scatchard analysis was carried out with crude or with purified c-IRP, the lower-affinity c-IRP site may represent contamination by n-IRP. The ^{14}C-IAA-n-IRP complex was reported to bind to coconut chromatin and to stimulate chromatin transcription by E. coli RNA polymerase two-fold. RNA synthesis supported by chick erythrocyte chromatin was unaffected. The model proposed, by analogy with steroid receptors, is that the high affinity c-IRP in chromatin acts as an acceptor site for the n-IRP-IAA complex to trigger specific gene transcription.

Superficially, the reported properties of the coconut receptors make them highly attractive candidates as genuine auxin receptors. Unfortunately, many of the claims made for n-IRP have only been outlined in conference proceedings (Biswas et al., 1975) and experimental details elsewhere are also often unsatisfactory. For example, amounts of starting material and recoveries cannot be deduced for either receptor, the auxin-specificity of c-IRP binding has not been examined at all, and the data for n-IRP (single point figures with only two compounds other than IAA) are inadequate. Nor does it appear that any compound other than IAA has been tested in relation to the reported effects on RNA synthesis. Other reservations have been expressed by Kende and Gardner (1976) and by Rubery (1981). No further publications on these proteins have appeared in recent years, and the exotic nature of the source material has so far inhibited independent evaluation.

5.4.2 Tobacco

In addition to the particulate sites discussed in section 5.3, the Leiden group has also investigated soluble (cytosolic) auxin-binding proteins from tobacco callus cultures. High affinity binding (K_d 10^{-8}M) was detected using high specific activity tritiated IAA and dextran-charcoal assay (Oostrom et al., 1975). The concentration of binding sites was consistently very low (ca. 0.01 pmol/mg protein = 0.01 pmol/g tissue). In common with the membrane-bound sites in tobacco, binding was time- and temperature-dependent (requiring 30 min. at 24-30°C), but with a higher pH optimum, pH 7.5-7.8 (Oostrom et al., 1980). The binding protein(s) were partially purified by gel permeation (giving an approximate molecular weight of 300,000 daltons) and by ion exchange chromatography. Affinity chromatography on 2,4-D coupled to aminohexyl-Sepharose was unsuccessful, doubtless because of the absence of a free carboxyl group. It would be of interest to try the 2,4-D-lysine adsorbent (Venis, 1971), since this does have a free (lysyl) carboxyl. Binding affinities of auxin analogues estimated from competitive displacement experiments (Table 5.10) were in reasonably good agreement with relative physiological activities (determined in other tissues). In addition, several inactive indolic compounds also failed to compete for IAA-^{3}H binding, though it would be instructive to have data for more closely related inactive or very weak auxins such as benzoic acid, phenoxyacetic acid, 2,6-D. As with the particulate binding sites, soluble binding activity may be developmentally regulated, since it was undetectable in crude extracts from freshly-excised or subcultured tissue and reached a maximum at 10-12 days after transfer, declining thereafter (Fig. 5.21). Bogers et al. (1980) raised the possibility that this temporal variation might reflect changes in a binding inhibitor rather than in receptor concentration, since they found that binding activity could be detected in fresh tissue if extracts were first passed through Sepharose. They did not, however, indicate whether activity in such partially-purified extracts changed with time after sub-culture.

Table 5.10 Comparative physiological activities and binding affinities for
tobacco soluble protein of a range of auxin analogues (from
Oostrom et al., 1980)

Compound	Auxin activity[a]	K_d (M)
IAA	+++	10^{-8}
NAA	+++	1.25×10^{-8}
2-NAA	+	10^{-7}
NOA	++	2.5×10^{-8}
2,4-D	+++	3.3×10^{-8}
3,5-D	0	No competition
2,4,5-T	+++	5.0×10^{-8}
2,4,5-TP[b]	0	10^{-6}
TIBA	Transport inhibitor	10^{-8}

[a] Measured in wheat or pea bioassays

[b] 2,4,5-trichlorophenoxy-n-propionic acid

Although Oostrom et al. (1980) could not improve binding activity by
including a proteolytic inhibitor or an adsorbent for phenolics, Van der
Linde et al. (1984) succeeded in enhancing binding protein yield with a
borate buffer extraction procedure that greatly reduced polyphenol
contamination. The active protein fraction obtained by this method eluted
from gel filtration columns in the 150,000-200,000 molecular weight range,
somewhat lower than the previous apparent value which may have been
magnified by polyphenol complexation. RNA synthesis by isolated tobacco
nuclei was stimulated by soluble auxin-binding protein in an IAA-dependent
manner (Table 5.11). It was not possible to evaluate the effect of the
receptor protein alone because of contamination by high nucleic acid-
independent nucleotide polymerase activity. The IAA-dependent stimulation
appeared to be of RNA polymerase II activity, since no stimulatory effect
was obtained in the presence of α-amanitin. Even with the improved
extraction procedure, binding activity of different preparations still
varied widely, from 0-0.2 pmol/mg protein. Enhanced RNA synthesis was only
observed when the receptor preparations showed detectable auxin-binding, but

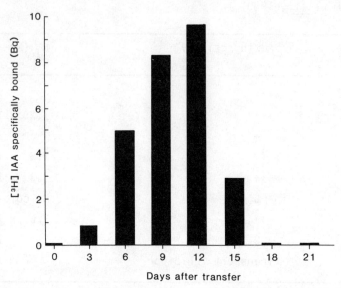

Fig. 5.21 - IAA binding by cytoplasmic proteins from tobacco callus after different periods of subculture (Oostrom et al., 1980)

Table 5.11   Stimulation of RNA synthesis in isolated tobacco nuclei by receptor fractions as a function of the IAA concentration. The receptor occupancy was calculated by using a K_d for IAA of 6.3×10^{-9}M (Van der Linde et al., 1984)

IAA concentration (M)	Receptor occupancy (%)	Stimulation (%)
10^{-9}	14	18
2.5×10^{-9}	29	16
10^{-8}	61	26
2.5×10^{-8}	80	31
10^{-6}	99	45

above this threshold there was no quantitative correlation between the two activities. Recent preliminary work reported at the 1984 FEBS Congress (Van der Linde et al., 1985) suggests that an important source of preparative variability may be receptor dephosphorylation, since conditions designed to minimise phosphatase activity and encourage phosphorylation led to greatly improved auxin-binding activity. Inactive preparations would be activated with ATP + Mg^{2+}. If confirmed, this will be the second plant receptor system in which phosphorylative control has been implicated, the first being the fusicoccin receptor (Aducci et al., 1984b). Moreover it should open the way for more detailed characterization of a promising system where progress has previously been hindered by problems of reproducibility.

5.4.3 Other systems

Likholat et al. (1974) reported that IAA added to the homogenization and wash media enhanced RNA synthesis by wheat coleoptile chromatin, but was without effect if added only to the in vitro reaction mixture. This finding is comparable to that of Matthysse and Phillips (1969) for nuclei (see Chapter 3). Binding of IAA-^{14}C by the cytosol fraction (detected by dextran-charcoal assay) was about five times higher in extracts from 36-hour-old, rather than from 72-hour-old, plants. These and other data on stimulation of chromatin RNA synthesis by membrane fractions incubated with IAA, were interpreted in terms of a transition of the auxin receptors from a 'soluble' to a membrane-bound state during passage of the cells from a dividing (36-hour) to an elongating (72-hour) phase. The membrane effects on RNA synthesis are somewhat similar to those described in soybean (see Chapter 3) by Hardin et al. (1972). Auxin binding by the wheat cytosol fraction was saturable upon addition of unlabelled IAA, but no attempt to estimate binding constants was made.

A charcoal adsorption assay (as well as non-equilibrium gel filtration) was also used by Ihl (1976) to study IAA binding to high speed supernatants from soybean cotyledons. However, most of the data were obtained by feeding IAA-^{14}C in vivo and there was no evidence to indicate that the label associated with the macromolecular fraction was still IAA, or that the binding was reversible in vitro. Similarly, binding saturation by unlabelled IAA or by other analogues was determined by feeding tissue 10^{-5}M IAA-^{14}C with or without a large excess (2.75 mM) of the cold compound. The observed reduction in macromolecular binding could therefore represent, amongst other things, competition for uptake.

Several reports of soluble auxin-binding proteins have appeared in which the assay method consisted of ammonium sulphate precipitation of a protein-labelled hormone mixture - from French bean (Wardrop and Polya, 1977), from peas (Jacobsen, 1982) and from mung beans (Sakai and Hanagata, 1983; Sakai, 1984). In addition, Murphy (1979) claimed that the auxin-binding properties of bovine serum albumin (BSA) would qualify it as an auxin receptor were it to be extracted from a plant. In all these cases, ammonium sulphate precipitation was the sole method of assay, but it has been found that this assay can be grossly misleading, generating interactions that are not detectable by more rigorous, homogeneous assays (Venis, 1984). For example, pea epicotyl protein prepared and assayed according to Jacobsen (1982) showed apparent auxin-binding activity, but none when assayed by equilibrium dialysis or by centrifugal ultrafiltration (Table 5.12). More recently, Jacobsen (1984) has claimed that the assay is valid because after isoelectric focussing not all of the protein fractions showed auxin-binding activity. Since proteins of different composition will vary in their hydrophobic interactions on unfolding, this finding is hardly surprising. A similar discrepancy between precipitation and equilibrium dialysis assays was observed with the French bean protein (Venis, 1984). Following their original report, Wardrop and Polya (1980) subsequently found that the bean protein co-purified with ribulose-1,5-bisphosphate carboxylase, and it does seem inherently improbable that the world's most abundant protein should be a hormone receptor. Auxin binding by BSA was confirmed (Venis, 1984), but activity was greatly reduced in equilibrium dialysis compared with precipitation assays, to a specific activity of around 1% of that found for purified NAA-binding proteins solubilized from maize membranes (Venis, 1980). On the other hand, the latter proteins were used to show that in some cases assay by ammonium sulphate precipitation can be a reliable guide to binding activity, provided that the assay is validated against one or more independent and unambiguous assays. Any reports without such confirmation must be treated with reserve.

As well as working with the membrane-bound sites in maize coleoptiles, Murphy (1980b) has shown that cytoplasmic fractions from the same tissues also have auxin-binding activity. Although this was determined by ammonium sulphate precipitation, preliminary studies (Venis, unpublished data) have shown that activity in these preparations is also readily detectable by

Table 5.12 Binding of NAA-^{14}C by pea epicotyl protein assayed by different procedures. All assays contained ca. 225 Bq ml^{-1} 5 x 10^{-5}M unlabelled NAA. The amount of protein per assay was 200 μg (precipitation assay) or 500 μg (equilibrium dialysis, ultrafiltration) in 50 mM Tris HCl pH 8.0 (Venis, 1984)

Assay method	NAA bound (Bq x 10^2)		
	^{14}C only	^{14}C + ^{12}C	Saturable
Precipitation	3948	2228	1720
Equilibrium dialysis	255	243	12
Ultrafiltration (MPS-1)	427	460	-33

equilibrium dialysis. In addition, Murphy (1980b) did have an independent check from purification studies in which the chromatographic columns were equilibrated and developed in NAA-^{14}C and binding fractions were detected by elevation of the radioactivity above the baseline level. In order to obtain satisfactory chromatography, it was necessary first to adsorb phenolics with dextran-charcoal. By gel permeation, the major auxin-binding region could then be located at 38,700 daltons, eluting slightly later than the solubilized membrane site (estimated at 43,700 daltons). Scatchard analysis revealed a single kinetic class of binding sites (K_d for NAA = 3.6 x 10^{-6}M; 160 pmol/g). On ion exchange and hydroxylapatite chromatography, however, the cytoplasmic binding activity was heterogeneous, whereas the membrane receptor protein still eluted as a single peak. Binding specificity was examined with a range of auxin analogues using both unfractionated cytoplasmic preparations and solubilized membrane sites. The correlation between auxin activity and binding activity appeared to be at least as good with the cytosol fraction as with the membrane sites or even better in some respects (Table 5.13). In particular the poor competition by PAA and phenylurea for cytosol-NAA-^{14}C binding, and the superior displacement by 2,4-D (relative to its effect on membrane site binding) are more in accord with the physiological activities of the compounds.

The characteristics of soluble binding in maize are sufficiently interesting to merit further investigation, but only this single report has appeared. In particular the specificity needs to be examined by another assay method to see if the correlations still hold. If so, the relationship, if any, of the soluble binding protein(s) to the membrane binding protein(s) of somewhat similar molecular weight would be an interesting area for study.

Table 5.13 Competition for NAA-^{14}C binding to cytoplasmic or solubilized membrane protein preparations from maize. Compounds tested at two concentrations; competition expressed as % of displacement caused by 10^{-4}M NAA. Assay by ammonium sulphate precipitation (from Murphy, 1980b)

Compound	Cytosol		Membrane	
	10^{-4}M	10^{-5}M	10^{-4}M	10^{-5}M
NAA	45	100	91	100
IAA	14	67	28	81
2,4,5-T	26	75	34	81
PAA	-2	25	80	94
Phenylurea	-4	15	24	71
NOA	17	58	9	45
2,4-D	23	80	11	57
Benzoic acid	<1	17	<1	12

6 Binding of Other Hormones and Regulators

6.1. CYTOKININS

There is overwhelming evidence (noted in Chapter 1) that the primary biological activity of cytokinins can be attributed to the free molecules per se rather than to incorporation into macromolecules. Nevertheless, given the occurrence of cytokinin bases in the anticodon region of certain tRNA molecules and an implied function in codon-anti-codon recognition, it is perhaps not surprising that cytokinin binding sites were first reported on ribosomes, from Chinese cabbage leaves (Berridge et al., 1970). However, this binding was of low affinity and hence of doubtful significance, though there seemed to be some correlation between biological activity of analogues and the molar binding ratio per ribosome. Ribosomal binding was re-examined by Fox and Erion (1975) in wheat germ and tobacco callus with lower labelled cytokinin concentrations than those used in the earlier work. This permitted the detection of a set of high affinity sites (K_d 6×10^{-7}M for BAP, benzyladenine), at a concentration of one binding site per ribosome, in addition to the low affinity binding (K_d $>10^{-4}$M) found previously. Rat liver and E. coli ribosomes also bound BAP-^{14}C, albeit substantially less than the plant ribosomes when compared at a single ligand concentration. Whether this binding is to similar sites present at lower concentrations, or to different sites of lower affinity is not clear. The high affinity sites could be removed from the ribosomes by washing with 0.5M KCl and this binding activity was recovered in the salt wash. It was non-dialysable and susceptible to heat and to trypsin treatment though not to ribonuclease, indicating the proteinaceous nature of the binding moiety.

The large majority of subsequent cytokinin binding studies have been carried out with source material similar or identical to that used by Fox and Erion (1975), i.e. wheat germ and tobacco. The wheat germ system is easily the best characterised biochemically, having been studied in several independent laboratories, though its function is still far from clear.

6.1.1. Wheat germ and allied sources

The ribosomal salt wash from the wheat germ preparations yielded a linear Scatchard plot, indicating that only the high affinity sites were present (Fox and Erion, 1977). An apparently identical binding protein, CBF-1, was also found in the cytosolic (ribosomal supernatant) fraction, at 2-3 times the amount associated with ribosomes. Subsequent studies, both by this group and others, have for the most part simply used low speed supernatants (<50,000g), that include ribosomes, as a starting point for purification. On the other hand, Erion and Fox (1981) have pointed out that the ribosomes act as a kind of affinity matrix for CBF-1 and the salt wash thus gives considerable initial purification. The apparent molecular weight of partially purified CBF-1 (gel filtration) was first reported as 93,000 daltons (Fox and Erion, 1977). Another binding fraction, CBF-2, was also found in cytosol preparations, but this was later regarded (Erion and Fox, 1981) as partly-degraded CBF-1. For the remainder of this section therefore, the generic abbreviation CBP will be used in referring to the predominant high-affinity cytokinin binding protein of wheat germ studied by several groups and originally designated CBF-1 by Fox and co-workers.

Subsequent investigations, from Fox's laboratory and elsewhere (Polya and Davis, 1978; Moore, 1979; Polya and Davies, 1983), have revised the gel filtration estimates of molecular weight upwards to varying extents. The overall picture appears somewhat confusing, as do the plethora of putative subunits derived from SDS polyacrylamide gels (Table 6.1). There is little doubt, despite differences in purification protocols, that the various groups are studying essentially the same protein, and it seems most probable that the discrepancies reflect varying degrees of proteolysis, though variable phosphorylation would be another factor (Polya and Davies, 1983). Indeed, Fox and Gregerson (1982) found differences in subunit composition of CBP derived from different samples of wheat germ, and the most recent evidence (Brinegar and Fox, 1985) suggests that CBP is actually a trimer of a single polypeptide type of 54,000 daltons. It was felt that the size heterogeneity previously observed derives from degradative effects of the milling process, since CBP isolated from excised mature wheat embryos showed only the 54,000 dalton polypeptide on SDS gels. When total protein extracts from immature embryos were run on gels, Western blotted and reacted with wheat germ CBP antiserum, predominantly the 54,000 dalton band was detected

116

(not lower mol. wt. bands), beginning at 20 days post-anthesis and
increasing thereafter. In addition there was reactivity towards a doublet at

Table 6.1 - Properties of cytokinin binding protein from wheat germ and
from barley embryos. n = number of binding sites per protein
molecule or (Fox and Erion, 1975) per ribosome

Reference	$K_d \times 10^{-6}M$	n	MW kilo-daltons	Subunits kilodaltons
Wheat germ				
Fox & Erion, 1975	0.6 (BAP)	1		
Fox & Erion, 1977	0.5 (BAP)	1	93	56,37
Erion & Fox, 1981	0.5 (BAP)	1	155	57,53,39,34
Brinegar & Fox, 1985			ca.160	54
Polya & Davis (1978)	0.2 (kinetin; pptn.assay) 7.5 (kinetin; equil.dial.)	1.7	180	60,46,43,14,13
Polya & Davies (1983)		1.1	140	60,42,37
Moore (1979)	1.2 (kinetin)	1.5	122	56,40,15
Barley embryo				
Reddy et al., 1983	0.66 (BAP)	1	155	57,53,39,36

66,000-68,000 daltons, which also appeared predominantly in immuno-
precipitates of immature embryo poly(A)RNA translation products. Whether or
not this polypeptide represents a precursor to the 54,000 dalton CBP
polypeptide remains to be established. Polya and Davies (1983) found that a
protein kinase in wheat germ phosphorylated CBP, predominantly their 60,000
dalton subunit plus low molecular weight polypeptides (16-18,000), while the
42,000 and 37,000 dalton subunits were very poorly labelled. This pattern

117

could be taken to support the suggestion of proteolysis of a single parent polypeptide. CBP phosphorylation was not activated by cytokinins.

CBP has generally been assayed by equilibrium dialysis, though Moore (1979) used non-equilibrium gel filtration and a DEAE filter assay. Polya and Davis (1978) used an ammonium sulphate precipitation procedure (Chapter 2) which is capable of generating artefactual binding (Chapter 5), but this was backed up by equilibrium dialysis and appears to have proved satisfactory for isolation purposes. However, the binding affinities estimated by the two methods differed by more than an order of magnitude (Table 6.1). In addition the precipitation assay indicated that binding was essentially independent of pH over the range pH 5.5-9.2, whereas Moore (1979) was able to detect an optimum at pH 6.6 by gel filtration assay, though the pH-activity profile was still fairly broad.

Both conventional (ion exchange, gel permeation) and affinity column procedures have been applied to CBP purification. After a series of gel filtration steps, Polya and Davis (1978) obtained a preparation in which cytokinin binding activity co-chromatographed precisely with a single peak of carbohydrate (5% by weight) and protein (Fig. 6.1). Since binding

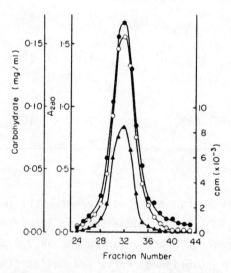

Fig. 6.1 - Final Sephacryl S-200 purification of wheat germ cytokinin binding protein. (▲) kinetin binding; (●) carbohydrate; (o) A_{280} (Polya and Davis, 1978)

activity was retained on a concanavalin A-Sepharose column and eluted by α-methylglucoside, CBP may well be glycosylated; other groups have not commented on carbohydrate content of CBP. Affinity chromatography has been based on periodate-oxidised cytokinin ribosides coupled either to aminohexyl-Sepharose (Moore, 1979) or to adipic acid dihydrazide-Sepharose (Erion and Fox, 1981). Bound CBP could not be efficiently eluted from either column with cytokinins, whereas urea was effective - but inconvenient - with both adsorbents. Moore (1979) found that the most useful strategy was to overload the column, after which CBP activity could be eluted as a sharp peak with pH 4 acetate. This method sacrifices more than half the total activity in the flow-through eluate, but since CBP is an abundant protein (see later), this factor is of no great consequence. Originally Erion and Fox (1981) showed an elution profile in which the bulk of CBP activity was removed under non-denaturing conditions with 2.5M KCl, giving 25-fold purification with 31% recovery, but subsequently (Fox and Gregerson, 1982) it was stated that high salt was ineffective and that 5M urea was necessary; the reason for this discrepancy is not apparent.

At saturation, there is about 1 molecule of cytokinin bound per CBP molecule (Table 6.1). Since there is also 1 cytokinin molecule bound per ribosome, there would seem to be 1 CBP molecule associated with each ribosome. The bulk of the CBP is in the cytosol and the ribosomal association could be a fortuitous in vitro relationship rather than functionally significant in vivo. Erion and Fox (1981) considered the stoichiometry to be more than coincidental and obtained a certain amount of supporting evidence from affinity chromatography and cross-linking experiments using intact and CBP-stripped ribosomes. If the ribosomal association does have any physiological relevance, it could conceivably be connected with recognition of cytokinin bases in tRNA, but it has been stated (Fox and Erion, 1977) that tRNA does not interact with CBP. Erion and Fox (1981) have also stated that the intact CBP molecule is needed for binding, and that isolated subunits, either singly or in various combinations, did not bind cytokinins - though this could simply reflect irreversible conformational alteration by SDS or urea. However, if in fact CBP consists of a trimer of identical subunits, then since there is only one cytokinin binding site per CBP molecule, it is likely that all subunits participate in formation of the binding domain.

The synthesis and biological activities of potential cytokinin photoaffinity reagents were reported by Theiler et al. (1976) and by Sussman and Kende (1977). However, the first attempt to examine the effectiveness of one of these compounds for its intended purpose was described by Mornet et al. (1979). They confirmed the earlier report (Theiler et al., 1976) that the 2-azido derivative of isopentenyladenine (i^6Ade) was somewhat more active than i^6Ade itself in a tobacco callus bioassay and also showed that 8-azido cytokinins were even more active (about ten-fold more active than the parent molecules), in general agreement with the data of Sussman and Kende (1977) for 8-azido-BAP. Nevertheless, for reasons not entirely clear it was the less active 2-azido-i^6Ade rather than the 8-azido analogue that was evaluated as a photoaffinity label. The compound competed with kinetin-^{14}C for binding to CBP (in the dark), while photolysis of 2-azido-i^6Ade in the presence of CBP resulted in nearly 80% reduction in subsequent kinetin-^{14}C binding, suggesting that the reagent binds at or near the active site. Keim and Fox (1980) similarly evaluated the corresponding 2-azido BAP, but in addition introduced ^{14}C at the methylene position to facilitate detection of covalent binding. The binding affinity for CBP (K_d 6.7x10^{-7}M) was very similar to that of the parent compound. When labelled 2-azido-BAP was photolyzed in the presence of CBP, radioactivity was incorporated into the protein, whereas there was little incorporation into an 'inert' protein (ovalbumin) under the same conditions (Fig. 6.2). Addition of a 3-fold excess of unlabelled BAP prior to photolysis reduced covalent incorporation by 40%, suggesting that the azido analogue labels, partly anyway, at or near the cytokinin binding site. However, the binding activity of CBP (using BAP-^{3}H) measured after photo-labelling with various concentrations of the ^{14}C-azido compound was reduced only by 28% even when 0.95 mol/mol protein of photoaffinity ligand was covalently bound. The curved Scatchard plot obtained with the modified CBP could not be unambiguously interpreted, but indicated that both binding affinity and site number may have been reduced. These data, plus the fact that the 2-position on cytokinins does not seem to be critically involved in ligand-protein interaction, suggested that the photoaffinity reagent may be labelling various amino acids at the periphery of the binding site and therefore only partly, and variably, occluding access by ligand. SDS gel electrophoresis of affinity-labelled CBP showed that all four subunits were labelled. Whilst labelling of dissimilar

subunits is not necessarily incompatible with a 1:1 cytokinin:CBP molar
binding ratio, the result is more readily interpretable if CBP in fact

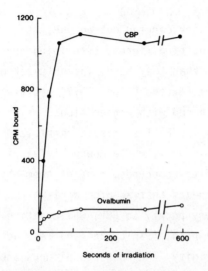

Fig. 6.2 - Photo-affinity labelling of wheat germ CBP with 2-azido-
6-benzylaminopurine -^{14}C, compared with ovalbumin labelling under the
same conditions (Keim and Fox, 1980)

consists of an oligomer of identical subunits (Brinegar and Fox, 1985)
susceptible to varying degrees of proteolysis.

Is wheat germ CBP a cytokinin receptor? Aside from the fact that its only
known biological property is an ability to bind cytokinins, there are two
main arguments against a receptor role. One relates to the abundance of the
protein, the other to its binding spectrum. CBP is present in wheat germ at
a very high concentration, estimated at 2.2-2.7 mg/g fresh wt. (Erion and
Fox, 1981; Polya and Davis, 1978) or about 20 nmol/g fresh wt. This is an
excessively high concentration for a receptor protein, not far from three
orders of magnitude higher than the concentrations of auxin- or NPA-binding
sites in maize coleoptiles for example (Chapters 4 and 5), and the maize
sites are themselves regarded as fairly abundant. Against this, Erion and
Fox (1981) have argued that the wheat embryo should be regarded as a storage
reservoir of CBP which quickly becomes diluted during germination by cell
division. They cite preliminary antibody evidence showing that immediately
upon germination the amount of CBP falls to a very low level and only rises

again during formation of the female reproductive tissues. This evidence remains unpublished, though a very similar claim (again unsupported) has also been made regarding a comparable barley protein (Reddy et al., 1983; see below).

Considering the amount of work carried out on CBP, it is surprising that the relative binding affinities of different cytokinins and analogues have not been examined rather more than they have. The only set of competitive displacement curves comes from Fox and Erion (1977) and these appear to be a mixed compilation of data obtained with either ribosomes or with partly purified CBP. Polya and Davis (1978) list displacement values for a range of compounds at two concentrations only, while Moore (1979) gives single concentration data for just five compounds, none of them physiologically inactive. Nevertheless, it appears that adenine derivatives with little or no cytokinin activity bind very poorly to CBP, while active 6-substituted adenines bind with reasonably high affinity and the less active ribosides with about ten-fold lower affinity. The most conspicuous anomaly, all groups are agreed, is the extremely low affinity of CBP for zeatin, the most active native cytokinin. Going beyond purines, Polya and Bowman (1979) have found that a wide variety of structurally dissimilar compounds can displace kinetin-^{14}C from CBP. Apart from herbicidal phenylureas, which might reasonably be expected to show some binding in view of the cytokinin activity of phenyl- and diphenylureas (Bruce and Zwar, 1966), these compounds included methylxanthines, triazines, carbamates, organotins, and a range of indoles. In many cases the interactions were shown to be competitive by double reciprocal analysis (e.g. Fig 6.2), with dissociation constants in the micromolar range (e.g. $9x10^{-7}$M for atrazine). The catholic nature of ligand binding to CBP would certainly seem to be a further strong argument against a receptor function. Erion and Fox (1981) have queried the significance of these data by suggesting that the CBP preparation was not homogeneous, but it seems to have been about as good as anyone else's (see Fig. 6.1 and original papers). A more pertinent comment might be that the data were all acquired with the ammonium sulphate precipitation assay, which magnifies hydrophobic interactions and can lead to artefactual binding. Thus in the earlier paper from Polya and Davis (1978), the apparent affinity of CBP for kinetin was much greater by precipitation assay than by equilibrium dialysis (Table 6.1). It would be of more than passing interest to know how the various non-purine compounds would behave in a non-precipitation assay.

Overall, however, the properties of CBP do not encourage the view that it is a cytokinin receptor. Rather, it may have a metabolic or sequestering role. If so, then as suggested by Polya and Bowman(1979), zeatin may in part owe its high biological activity to the very fact of its low affinity for non-receptor binding proteins such as CBP or analogous molecules.

Other cereal grains (barley, oat, rye) appear to contain cytokinin-binding proteins related immunochemically (Keim et al., 1981) and in other general properties to the wheat germ protein (Fox and Gregerson, 1982). Reddy et al. (1983) reported the isolation from barley embryos of a protein with very similar characteristics to wheat germ CBP (Table 6.1). It was claimed that the level of this protein increases during embryogenesis and falls to a very low level during germination, a claim similar to that made for wheat germ CBP. Remarkably, the barley protein was purified to apparent homogeneity by a single affinity column step following an ammonium sulphate cut (Fig. 6.3). Even more remarkably, the affinity adsorbent consisted of BAP coupled directly to CNBr-activated Sepharose with no spacer arm, and sharp elution was achieved without resort to extremes of pH or to chaotropic agents. In all, this represents an affinity chromatography ideal that is seldom realised, and it would be of interest to see if those working with

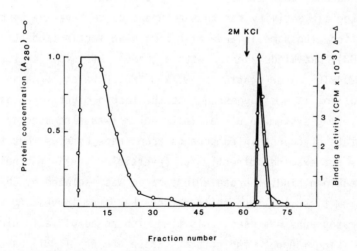

Fig. 6.3 - Benzyladenine-Sepharose 6B affinity chromatography of barley embryo CBP (Reddy et al., 1983)

wheat germ CBP can effect similar purification. It is possible that the steric hindrance introduced by omitting a spacer group lowers column affinity for CBP just sufficiently to permit efficient elution while retaining useful capacity.

6.1.2. Tobacco cells and other systems

The same affinity column had been used earlier by Takegami and Yoshida (1975) to isolate a low molecular weight (4000 dalton) cytokinin-binding polypeptide from tobacco leaves, but salt elution was ineffective in this case and 0.1 N KOH was used - a somewhat drastic measure. As with wheat germ CBP, this material was found both in the soluble fraction and in salt washes of ribosomes, but the large difference in molecular weight and the apparent inability of CBP fragments to bind cytokinins renders any relationship between the two proteins improbable. A glycopeptide of similar size (6000 daltons) that binds cytokinins (as well as IAA, tryptophan and Ca^{2+}) has been found in the cell wall-membrane matrix of the water mould Achlya (Le John, 1975). The tobacco leaf polypeptide was able to bind to 40S but not to 60S ribosomal subunits, and this binding was stimulated by BAP, optimally at 10^{-5}M (Takegami and Yoshida, 1977). It was suggested that it might be a subunit of an initiation factor and may have a role in mediating cytokinin effects on protein synthesis. However, the binding affinity (K_d $4x10^{-5}$M for BAP-^{14}C; Yoshida and Takegami, 1977) really seems too low in relation to cytokinin biological activity for this polypeptide to have any sort of receptor function. The same is true of a lima bean lectin (Roberts and Goldstein, 1983) that binds adenine with a greater affinity (K_d $1.2x10^{-5}$M) than BAP (K_d $2.4x10^{-5}$M) or zeatin (K_d $9.1x10^{-5}$M). However, because of its high concentration, it was suggested that the lectin might serve as a cytokinin buffering system. A BAP affinity column was also used by Harada (1980) to isolate glycoprotein components from grape berries, but the fractions were not examined directly for reversible cytokinin binding.

Another cytokinin binding protein in tobacco was isolated by Chen et al. (1980), but from tissue culture cells rather than from leaves. Again, affinity chromatography was used, this time with an adipic acid dihydrazide spacer arm, linking i^{6}Ado to the column. (Erion and Fox (1981) used similar coupling, but with BAP). Binding activity was eluted as a sharp peak with 1M KCl in pH 8 buffer and on gel filtration this material was resolved into a low affinity, heat-stable 123,000 dalton protein and a glycoprotein of 8500 daltons showing partially heat-sensitive, high affinity binding of i^6-Ade-^{3}H (K_d 8.8x10^{-7}M), with 2.1 binding sites per molecule. Other active cytokinins were bound with similar affinities (zeatin with rather lower affinity), while adenine did not bind. The common source species and similar low molecular size suggest a relationship between this protein and the tobacco leaf protein of Takegami and Yoshida (1975); further, both show time-dependent binding, requiring 1-2 hours incubation. The higher binding affinity of the tissue culture protein may be more apparent than real, since these data were obtained exclusively with the ammonium sulphate precipitation assay, which can lower apparent cytokinin K_d values about 40-fold (Table 6.1). This would bring the K_d in line with the Takegami and Yoshida (1975) figure for the tobacco leaf protein of 4x10^{-5}M, obtained by non-equilibrium gel filtration. Unless the tissue culture protein is found to retain its apparently higher affinity in a non-precipitation assay, it seems unlikely to be a receptor.

Cultured tobacco cells also contain particulate binding sites for cytokinins, sedimentable at 80,000g (Sussman and Kende, 1978). Using high specific activity BAP-^{3}H, a minor class of heat-labile, high affinity sites was found against a much larger background of low affinity, heat-stable binding (Fig. 6.4). Binding specificity was examined in a much more

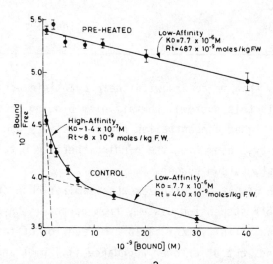

Fig. 6.4 - Scatchard plot of BAP-^{3}H binding to a particulate fraction from cultured tobacco cells (Sussman and Kende, 1978)

systematic way than usual, using a series of BAP analogues differing only in halogenation at various positions in the benzene ring, but embracing a wide range of cytokinin activity. High affinity binding (measured as displacement of 5nM BAP-^{3}H by 500 nM unlabelled compound) showed excellent correlation with cell division activity in the same tissue (Table 6.2). Binding of

Table 6.2 - High affinity binding and biological activities of halobenzyl BAP analogues in tobacco cell suspensions (from Sussman and Kende, 1978)

Substituent	Saturable binding (cpm)	Cell division activity
None (BAP)	318	+++
2-F	279	+++
'3-F	249	+++
4-F	271	+++
2-Cl	227	++
3-Cl	118	+
4-Cl	72	Inactive
2-Br	200	++
4-Br	34	Inactive

kinetin and zeatin was also in accord with their cytokinin activities (greater for kinetin in this system). Low affinity binding on the other hand, measured over a higher concentration range, was very poorly correlated with biological activity, resembling the binding spectrum obtained with a non-biological material, talcum powder.

Particulate binding of BAP-^{14}C with somewhat similar characteristics was detected in another cell suspension system, from carrot (Kobayashi et al., 1981). Again, both high affinity (K_d 3.3×10^{-8} M) and low affinity (K_d 6.4×10^{-6}M) sites were found, but at a lower abundance (1.1 pmol and 44 pmol/g respectively) than in tobacco cells. In competitive displacement experiments the order of effectiveness of different compounds was BAP>kinetin>zeatin>

i^6Ade>Ade; affinities of ribosides were mostly lower than the free bases. However, relative cytokinin activities in the carrot suspension system were not shown. Moreover, it is difficult to see how the kinetics of the low abundance, high affinity binding sites could be determined with any certainty with BAP-^{14}C whose specific activity was about 200-fold less than that of the BAP-^{3}H used by Sussman and Kende (1978). Calculation suggests that with the concentration of BAP-^{14}C used (10^{-8}M) and the amount of tissue per assay (1 g), not more than 30 dpm would be bound to high affinity sites and available for displacement. (Note also that in Figs. 1 and 2 of the paper the ordinate values should be divided by 3600; Reinert, personal communication).

Bud formation in moss protonemata is induced by cytokinin bases, the ribosides being very much less active. Binding of BAP-^{3}H to particulate fractions from _Funaria_ protonemata was studied by Gardner et al. (1978), and a reasonable correlation between cytokinin activity in bud induction and ability to displace BAP-^{3}H was found. However, kinetic analysis of binding saturation did not reveal a discrete set of high affinity sites, displacement being linearly related to log [BAP] over 4 orders of magnitude. This binding resembled, though differed in detail from, the characteristics of binding to talc. Potentially, this experimental material provides a useful cytokinin target system for receptor studies, but it seems that different approaches, perhaps by affinity labelling, are needed. Another potential target system, studied by Chung et al. (1979) is the dioecious plant _Mercurialis annua_, in which production of male flowers is controlled by cytokinins. Ribosomes from male flower buds contained about twice as many BAP binding sites as those from female buds, though with similar affinities (ca. 3×10^{-6}M). Although the magnitude of binding measured was fairly small (100-150 cpm saturable binding/assay), the displacement curves were of interest in indicating, uniquely for cytokinin-binding systems, a much higher affinity for zeatin (K_d ca. 2×10^{-7}M). This system does not appear to have been studied further.

Evidently no compelling candidate for a cytokinin receptor emerges from the various investigations that have been made. Wheat germ CBP is by far the best characterised, but has doubtful receptor status, for reasons discussed. The binding sites with the most appropriate properties in terms of affinity and specificity are the high affinity particulate sites in tobacco culture

cells (Sussman and Kende, 1978). However, these have not been characterised
further, perhaps because of the problems caused by the large excess of low
affinity, non-specific sites. Cytokinin photoaffinity labels have been
available for some time, but do not appear to have been successfully applied
to this system; the reagent would need to be tritiated to high specific
activity to be of much value for isolation and purification purposes.

6.2. GIBBERELLINS

The structural affinities between gibberellins and steroids, and their
common early biosynthetic steps, have directed thinking about gibberellin
receptors along animal steroid hormone lines, i.e. the cytoplasmic
receptor-nuclear translocation model. Since the steroid model is currently
undergoing an agonising reappraisal (see Chapter 1.1.), a rethink on
gibberellin receptors may be appropriate, directing effort at nuclear rather
than cytoplasmic fractions. In this section, attempts to detect soluble
binding will first be considered, followed by studies on gibberellin
associations with particulate fractions.

The gibberellin-responsive dwarf pea has been a favoured experimental
material. Several early unsuccessful attempts to detect binding in vitro
have been summarised by Kende and Gardner (1976). Subsequently both Stoddart
et al. (1974) and later Keith and Srivastava (1980), using high specific
activity GA_1-^3H, detected protein associations after feeding in vivo. In the
former work, epicotyls were supplied with GA_1-^3H for 12 hours at $25^{o}C$ and
the 20,000g supernatant fractionated by gel filtration. In addition to the
major peak of low mol. wt. (LMW) material, two peaks of radioactivity were
found associated with high (HMW) and intermediate (IMW) fractions (Fig.
6.5). These contained unchanged GA_1, whereas in the LMW fraction more than
60% GA_8, a major metabolite of GA_1 in dwarf pea, was found. This indicated
that the macromolecular fractions did not bind the inactive (and 2-
hydroxylated) GA_8, but then neither a receptor nor a GA_1 hydroxylase would
be expected to bind the product of the reaction. Since the extract was only
centrifuged at 20,000g, the HMW fraction will undoubtedly have contained
microsomes and ribosomes as well as soluble protein; indeed Keith and
Srivastava (1980) found that both ^3H and protein in this fraction were
reduced by about half after centrifugation at 100,000g x 1 hour. Both groups
found that much less GA_1-^3H was bound per unit fresh weight in the non-

128

responsive basal region of the epicotyl than in the responsive apical region (Fig. 6.5), but since the protein content was also lower there was little

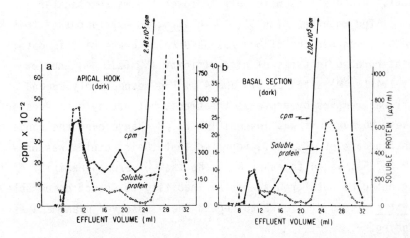

Fig. 6.5 - Sephadex G-200 elution profiles of supernatant fractions prepared from dwarf pea epicotyls allowed to imbibe GA_1-^{3}H for 12 hours in the dark. (a) Apical hooks or (b) Basal sections excised and homogenised. (Stoddart et al., 1974)

difference in specific activity. From in vivo feeding with two further GA_1-^{3}H analogues, the inactive 3-epi-GA_1 appeared not to bind to either HMW or IMW fractions (Stoddart et al., 1974), whereas 16-keto-GA_1 (originally regarded as inactive, but subsequently stated to have moderate activity in the dwarf pea bioassay; Keith and Srivastava, 1980) bound to both. It was possible to detect some binding of ^{3}H-GA_1 in vitro to unlabelled HMW and IMW fractions by equilibrum dialysis, but no information on saturability or site concentration was presented. This binding was about 70% exchangeable with excess unlabelled GA_1 in 1 hour and would therefore seem to be different in kind from the quantitatively much greater in vivo binding, which both groups found to be largely non-exchangeable.

Keith and Srivastava (1980) were able to repeat the observations of Stoddart et al. (1974) using the original conditions, but most of their work was carried out by feeding thin epicotyl sections (0.5-1 mm) with GA_3 at $0^{o}C$ for 3 days. The objective was to minimise metabolism and hope to simulate an in vivo equilibrium dialysis system. Gel filtration of supernatants obtained from $0^{o}C$ treatments again gave HMW and IMW peaks of bound GA_1, with mol.

I29

wts. very similar to those estimated by Stoddart et al. (1974). Although bound GA_1-^3H was not exchangeable in vitro either by GA_1, GA_3 or GA_8, active but not inactive gibberellins were able to lower the macromolecular associations if fed together with GA_1-^3H in vivo. An experiment of this kind with different concentrations of GA_1 was used to generate kinetic data, which were interpreted in terms of high affinity (K_d $6x10^{-8}M$) and low affinity (K_d $1.4x10^{-6}M$) sites at 0.5 and 4 pmol/g respectively. Bound radioactivity was removed by protease treatment, but not by nucleases or phospholipases. However, it was insensitive to pH change over the range pH 3-10 (though Stoddart et al., 1974 reported that their complex was only stable at pH 6-7.5). Taken together with the lack of exchangeability of in vivo binding noted by both groups and the inability to detect comparable binding in vitro, it is difficult to regard these observed phenomena as receptor binding.

Konjevic et al. (1976) also used peas (Alaska, a tall cultivar) as experimental material and attempted to examine binding in vitro. After crude homogenates were incubated with GA_3-^{14}C at room temperature for 30 min., an excluded peak of radioactivity was detected on gel filtration of a 100,000g supernatant. This could be resolved into several peaks by ion exchange chromatography, sucrose gradient centrifugation, or agarose electrophoresis. Over 90% of the 'bound' radioactivity was extractable by ethanol, but its chemical identity was not established, which is unfortunate, given the incubation conditions used. Both GA_{4+7} and the inactive GA_{13} reduced binding when pre-incubated with supernatant, and no data on saturability with GA_3 were presented. With the extremely low specific activity GA_3-^{14}C used, the chemical concentration in the incubations was $1.6x10^{-5}M$, and it seems unlikely that physiologically meaningful binding would be detectable under these conditions.

The in vivo equilibrium dialysis principle was further applied by Keith et al. (1980), to study putative GA_1 binding in barley aleurone layers. After incubating aleurones in ^3H-GA_1 for 72 hours at temperatures of 0.5-1.5^oC, no metabolism of the hormone was detectable. At this time the internal concentration of radioactivity exceeded that in the incubation medium, and this retention was reduced if excess unlabelled GA_1 was included during incubation, whereas the same concentration of the inactive GA_8 was without effect. Part of the observed retention was attributed to binding to gibberellin receptors, but no attempts to detect macromolecular association of the label were presented. Jelsema et al. (1977) had reported $GA_1-{}^3H$ binding to wheat aleurone grains, but saturable binding was less than 5% of the total and was not characterised.

The only convincing demonstration of exchangeable gibberellin binding in vitro has been by Keith et al. (1981, 1982), using 100,000g supernatants from cucumber hypocotyls. Binding of $GA_4-{}^3H$ was determined in the first paper by non-equilibrium gel filtration (also by equilibrium dialysis) and later by a more rapid DEAE-cellulose filter disc method. After subtraction of non-specific binding a single class of binding sites was found (K_d $7x10^{-8}M$), present at the very low concentration of 0.7 pmol/g fresh wt. On a specific activity (i.e. per mg protein) basis, binding was similar in the GA-responsive apical hook and in the non-responsive basal hypocotyl region. There was a very good correlation between the ability of analogues to displace $GA_4-{}^3H$ from the binding sites and their biological activities (Table 6.3). Subsequent double reciprocal analysis showed that inhibition by active GAs was competitive. Detection of $GA_1-{}^3H$ binding by extracts from

Table 6.3 - Displacement of $GA_4-{}^3H$ binding ($1.55 \times 10^{-8}M$) to cucumber hypocotyl soluble protein by unlabelled gibberellins (1.55×10^{-6}).
100% value = 5700 dpm/mg protein (from Keith et al., 1981)

	Binding, % of maximum	Gibberellin activity
$GA_4-{}^3H$ (control)	100	
+GA_1	44	++
+GA_3	33	++
+GA_4	28	+++
+GA_5	65	+
+GA_7	30	++++
+GA_8	72	None
+Keto GA_1	79	+
+Iodo GA_1-Me	72	None
+GA_{26}	91	None

GA-responsive maize second leaf sheaths has been noted in a preliminary abstract (Keith et al., 1984). These are encouraging reports, and the presence of binding sites in both responsive and non-responsive tissue need not necessarily be of concern, as discussed in Chapter 1.4. However, a note of caution has been sounded by Stoddart (1982) with the observation that the binding specificity also approximates to what one might expect of 2-hydroxylase substrates and that in general, gibberellin binding of one sort or another is seen in tissues that metabolise gibberellins readily, whereas in those that do not, but which are nevertheless highly responsive (e.g. lettuce hypocotyl), binding cannot be detected. Clearly, only further purification and characterisation will resolve this issue, but it should not be long before the suggestion can be tested with a purified 2-hydroxylase.

A very different kind of cellular gibberellin association has been examined in lettuce hypocotyls by Stoddart (1979 a,b) and Stoddart and Williams (1979, 1980). After hypocotyl sections were incubated in GA_1-^3H for varying periods (0.5-48 hours), the bulk of the tissue radioactivity was found in the 100,000g supernatant; of this only about 0.2% was macromolecular on gel filtration and the soluble fraction was not examined further. Between 5-20% of the tissue label was associated with cell-wall-containing material sedimenting at 2000g (2KP fraction), in a form that was largely or wholly resistant to repeated washing, to sedimentation through sucrose, electrophoresis, and to treatment with salt, organic solvents, cellulase or protease. This labelling increased linearly with time, was only slowly and partially removed by prolonged chasing (up to 33 hours) in unlabelled GA_1, and did not saturate with respect to GA_1 concentration over an extended range ($10^{-7}-10^{-3}M$). Incorporation was greatly reduced in disrupted tissue and was sensitive to inhibitors of protein synthesis. The general characteristics of this incorporation strongly suggest covalent linkages with components of the 2KP fraction. Digestion with 1M KOH (25-37°C, 8-12 hours) released the major part of the label, and on gel exclusion chromatography this appeared in two peaks, the larger one being associated with carbohydrate and of slightly greater molecular size than GA_1. Incorporation into 2KP material was highly correlated with growth rate. However, from kinetic studies carried out at 5°C and at 30°C it was concluded that the association either preceded the growth or was unconnected, but was not simply a consequence thereof (Stoddart and

Williams, 1980). It was speculated that attachment of gibberellins to sites in the cell wall might interfere with the activity of enzymes whose action leads to formation of growth-limiting wall linkages. As a suggested mode of action, this is clearly at odds with orthodox concepts of hormone action, which is no bad thing in itself. However, given that other gibberellin-specific effects (e.g. hydrolase induction in aleurones) almost certainly involve non-covalent hormonal attachment, it seems somewhat unlikely that fundamentally different modes of primary interaction would have developed for the same structurally-defined class of growth regulator.

Evidently all these systems are very far from being established as putative gibberellin receptors. The work of Keith et al. (1981, 1982) with cucumber extracts is perhaps the most promising, though the reservations expressed by Stoddart (1982) need to be addressed. At present, only the rudiments of the system have been studied, and even if the hydroxylase hurdle is cleared, there is still a long way to go to establish any sort of model, steroidal or otherwise. Interestingly, a recent abstract (Janik and Adler, 1984) reports the presence in Gladiolus ovules of an estradiol receptor with characteristics very similar to those in mammalian target cells. The protein is stated to translocate from cytoplasm to nucleus when activated by estradiol and to sediment at 4.7S in the activated form. The K_d was 1.1 nM and binding capacity around 4 pmol/g tissue, divided about equally between cytoplasm and nucleus. Estradiol, estriol and diethylstilbestrol bound, while testosterone and progesterone did not. Binding activity was not detected in anthers. Until experimental details appear, it is difficult to comment on these claims, except to note the remarkable parallelism with the (now slightly tarnished) classic animal steroid model. If substantiated in some form or another, this report will obviously be of considerable interest, not least because of the long-standing efforts to implicate steroidal substances in processes of floral initiation and sex expression. In addition, it could establish the possibility in plants of the sort of hormone action model that has been envisaged for gibberellins.

6.3. ABSCISIC ACID

Until recently only one solitary report on ABA binding had appeared, that of Hocking et al. (1978), who obtained saturable binding of ABA-^{3}H to membranous preparations from Vicia faba leaves. Greatest binding was found in a sucrose gradient fraction that was thought to be enriched in plasma membrane. Scatchard analysis suggested the presence of two classes of binding site, the higher affinity site having a K_d of 35nM, and an abundance of 3.5 pmol/g of tissue. No further information was given, nor has materialised since, and attempts to repeat this work using much higher specific activity ABA have been unsuccessful (R. Horgen, personal communication).

However, a dramatic advance has been made by Hornberg and Weiler (1984), who appear to have succeeded in photoaffinity labelling an ABA receptor in guard cells of Vicia faba. ABA contains an α,β-unsaturated ketone and such moieties can be photoactivated at around 330 nm; this principle has been used many times in the past, for example to photolabel ecdysterone receptors on Drosophila chromosomal puffs (Gronemeyer and Pongs, 1980). The ABA work rested on two further important considerations: firstly, the ability to obtain both labelled and unlabelled (+)ABA and (-)ABA by resolution of the enantiomers on immunoaffinity columns (Mertens et al., 1982); secondly, the fact that over a short period at any rate, stomatal closure in V. faba is induced only by the (+) enantiomer of ABA, so that labelling with (-)ABA provides an excellent control. Protoplasts were first incubated in ABA-^{3}H in the dark, then washed, irradiated and the amount of fixed label determined. Labelling of guard cell protoplasts was about 10-fold greater than that of mesophyll protoplasts, and in both types of cell there was a marked selectivity for the active (+) enantiomer (Fig. 6.6). Labelling of guard cell protoplasts showed saturation with increasing (+)ABA-^{3}H concentration, and addition of unlabelled (+)ABA prior to photolysis (but not (-)ABA) competed with (+)ABA-^{3}H for photo-induced covalent attachment (Fig. 6.7). From such data, the K_d of guard cell protoplast sites for (+)ABA was estimated at 3-4 nM, in good agreement with the concentration for half-maximal stomatal closure, ca. 5 nM. Since the protoplasts are washed prior to photoactivation, the rate of dissociation from the sites is evidently not too rapid, and this must make an important contribution to selectivity of labelling.

Brief (10 min.) trypsin treatment of the protoplasts left them intact, but completely abolished their subsequent ability to bind ABA-^{3}H, suggesting that the binding proteins are located on the external face of the plasma

membrane. SDS gels of guard cell protoplast lysates after photolabelling
revealed three bands A, B and C (mol. wt. 20,200; 19,300; 14,300

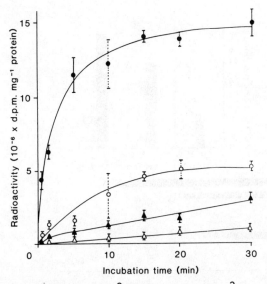

Fig. 6.6 - Kinetics of (+)ABA-^{3}H (●) or (-)ABA-^{3}H (o) binding to <u>V. faba</u>
guard cell protoplasts after UV irradiation. Triangles denote equivalent
experiment with mesophyll protoplasts (Hornberg and Weiler, 1984)

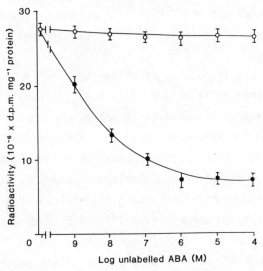

Fig. 6.7 - Competition by (+)ABA (●) or (-)ABA (o) with (+)ABA-^{3}H for
photoaffinity labelling of <u>V. faba</u> guard cell protoplasts
(Hornberg and Weiler, 1984)

respectively) that were clearly labelled (Fig. 6.8) and to a much greater extent than in lysates from mesophyll protoplasts. As the pH during

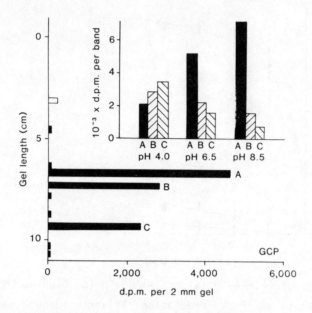

Fig. 6.8 - SDS-PAGE of photoaffinity-labelled guard cell protoplast proteins after incubation in (+)ABA-^{3}H at pH 6.5. Inset: Radioactivity recovered from bands A,B and C after incubation of guard cells with (+)ABA-^{3}H at different pH values (Hornberg and Weiler, 1984)

protoplast incubation was increased, labelling of one band increased, while the other two showed reduced labelling (Fig. 6.8). It was therefore suggested that there may be three distinct ABA-binding proteins, one (A) for ABA' and the other two for ABA-H, and that this would account for the ability of ABA to induce stomatal closure over an extended pH range. Finally, an excellent correlation was obtained between the activity of ABA analogues and related compounds in inducing stomatal closure in epidermal strips, and their ability to compete with (+)ABA-^{3}H binding to guard cell protoplasts.

This impressive piece of work satisfies, in a single paper, most of the criteria expected of a hormone receptor (Chapter 1.4.), including the all-important one of correlation of binding with a biological response. Reversible, non-covalent attachment of ABA to unmodified receptors remains to be established, but will doubtless follow. The calculated binding site concentration in target cells is very high (1.9×10^6 sites per guard cell), but given the likely difficulty of obtaining such cells in gram quantities, it may prove more rewarding for receptor isolation purposes to use non-target cells, since the lower site concentration will be more than offset by very much greater accessibility. Alternatively, provided that a screening assay can be developed, it may be possible to raise monoclonal antibodies to ABA receptors using membranes from lysed (guard cell) protoplasts, and then use these for receptor isolation by immunoaffinity chromatography. The way would then be open to probe for ABA receptors in other responsive tissues, many of which do not appear to distinguish between the enantiomers of ABA.

6.4. ETHYLENE

At first sight the technical problems in determining equilibrium binding of a labelled gaseous hormone seem formidable. However, ethylene binding sites are now being actively investigated by two separate groups whose efforts have been greatly facilitated by the fact that the ethylene-binding site complexes so far discovered have very slow rates of dissociation (and association), enabling them to be studied by non-equilibrium methods. This work was initiated independently and more or less simultaneously in the laboratories of Sisler (Raleigh) and Hall (Aberystwyth). In the latter case it arose out of the discovery that ethylene partitions into many plant tissues to a very much greater extent than would be expected from the normal air/water partition coefficient (Jerie et al., 1978, 1979). In Vicia faba it was found that this phenomenon reflected oxidation to ethylene oxide (discussed later), while in Phaseolus vulgaris compartmentation was due to the presence of high affinity binding sites for ethylene. Fractions from crude P. vulgaris cotyledon extracts separated on sucrose gradients were found to bind ethylene-^{14}C (overnight incubation, 25°C) and the same gradient distribution of activity was found if the cotyledons were pre-labelled with ethylene in vivo (Bengochea et al., 1980a). Both the in vitro assay (which involves venting off unbound ethylene after incubation) and the pre-labelling method were possible only because of the very slow rate of ethylene dissociation from the binding site, noted above. The K_d (after correction to infinite site dilution) was calculated at 0.1 nM in solution (Bengochea et al., 1980b), with 3-40 pmol of binding sites/g tissue, the number tending to increase with cotyledon age, in accordance with observations of Jerie et al. (1979) in intact cotyledons. The ratio of the rate constants of dissociation and association (K_{-1}/K_1) were in good agreement with the equilibrium K_d value. Structural analogues competitively inhibited ethylene binding (Fig. 6.9), and the order of activity closely paralleled relative physiological effectiveness (Bengochea et al., 1980b).

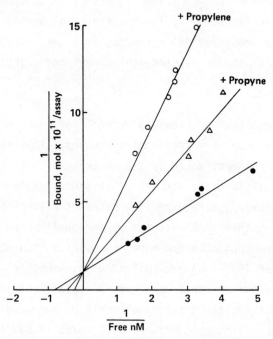

Fig. 6.9 - Double reciprocal plots of ethylene $-^{14}C$ binding to cell-free preparations from P. vulgaris cotyledons in the presence or absence of competitors (Bengochea et al., 1980b)

On isopycnic centrifugation three bands of binding activity were seen (Fig. 6.10) and from comparison with marker enzyme distributions these were provisionally assigned to protein body membranes and ER, and perhaps also to a fraction of the plasma membrane (Evans et al., 1982a). General support for these conclusions was provided from localisation of binding sites by light and electron microscope autoradiography, made possible by the slow dissociation behaviour and the ability of osmium to form an insoluble complex with ethylene (Evans et al., 1982b).

The binding sites in P. vulgaris cotyledons could be solubilised from
96,000g pellets using Triton X-100, yielding preparations whose general

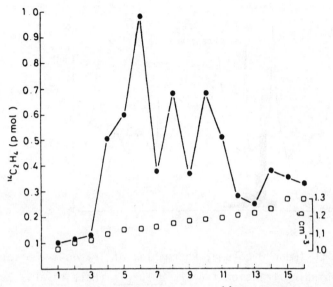

Fig. 6.10 - Distribution of ethylene -^{14}C binding activity after
isopycnic centrifugation of P. vulgaris particulate preparations
(Evans et al., 1982a)

properties in terms of affinity, site concentration, and analogue
competition were very similar to those observed in the membrane-bound system
(Thomas et al., 1984). Significant changes were the even slower rates of
association and dissociation, a shift in pH optimum from 7.5-9.5 (in the
membranes) to around pH 5, and a greater resistance of the solubilised sites
to proteolysis. Some or all of these changes may have been connected with
shielding of the protein molecules by detergent, a supposition supported by
the failure to precipitate the binding activity in its isoelectric region
(pH 3-5) or with ammonium sulphate (Thomas et al., 1985). The ethylene-
binding protein appears to be strongly hydrophobic and asymmetric, with a
mol. wt. in the range 52,000-60,000 daltons. Purification has been hampered
by the shielding effects arising from the need to maintain the presence of
detergent, though slight purification was effected by various means (Thomas
et al., 1985). However, preliminary findings (Hall et al., 1984) indicate
that far more effective purification can be achieved by FPLC (Fast Protein

Liquid Chromatography) on a Mono Q (Pharmacia) anion exchange column (Fig. 6.11).

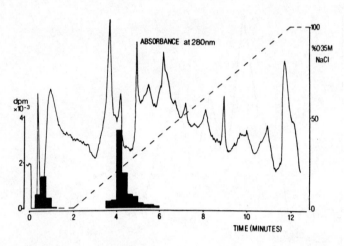

Fig. 6.11 - FPLC (Mono Q column, Pharmacia) of Triton X-100 solubilised ethylene-binding fraction from P. vulgaris (Hall et al., 1984)

Sisler has used an in vivo method to examine ethylene binding by tobacco leaves (Sisler, 1979; Goren and Sisler, 1984) and by leaves and other tissues of a wide range of species (Sisler, 1982b; Goren and Sisler, 1984; Sisler et al., 1985). This involves exposing tissue to ethylene-^{14}C in a desiccator until equilibrium is reached and then rapidly transferring the tissue to another vessel in which bound ethylene is released, trapped in mercuric perchlorate and counted for radioactivity. A broadly similar procedure was also used to measure binding in vitro, predominantly with mung bean preparations (Sisler, 1980, 1982a; Beggs and Sisler, 1985) but also in extracts from tomato fruit (Sisler, 1982b) and from a wide range of seeds (Sisler, 1984). The accumulated data from both laboratories (Table 6.4) reveal a close similarity between K_d values and site concentrations (n), except that French bean (Phaseolus vulgaris) cotyledons appear to contain rather more binding sites than the other species, while the concentration in tomato fruits is extremely low. The seed data of Sisler (1984) were only briefly documented, as dpm/g values, but suggested that seeds of some other species (e.g. mung bean, azuki bean) may be better sources of ethylene-binding sites than P. vulgaris. Affinities for analogues are also

Table 6.4 - Kinetic properties of ethylene binding systems. For comparative
purposes all K_d values refer to gas phase concentrations,
without corrections to infinite site dilution.
N.D. = not determined.

Source		K_d (gas) nM	n pmol/g	Reference
French bean:	membrane preps. (cotyledons)	3.6-8.2	3-40	Bengochea et al., 1980a
	: solubilized preps. (cotyledons)	1.7-5.0	32-34	Thomas et al., 1984
	: leaves	8.9	2.0	Goren and Sisler, 1985
Tobacco	: leaves	12	3.5	Sisler, 1979
Carnation	: petals	4.5	6.0	Sisler et al., 1985
	: leaves	4.0	2.0	" " "
Pineapple	: leaves	7.6	5.7	Goren and Sisler, 1985
Japanese privet:	leaves	14	6.8	Goren and Sisler, 1985
Mung bean	: solubilized preps. (shoots)	13	N.D.	Sisler, 1982a
	: " " "	4.5	N.D.	Beggs and Sisler, 1985
Tomato	: leaves	13	2.0	Sisler, 1982b
	: fruit (solubilised preps.)	13	0.07	" "

generally similar between the better-studied systems and in line with
relative physiological activities, apart from ethylene antagonists. In
cell-free systems, cycloalkene antagonists of ethylene action (e.g.
2,5-norbornadiene) bind much less effectively to French bean preparations

than to those from mung bean (see Smith and Hall, 1985, for a tabulated comparison of analogue data. It should be noted that Sisler habitually uses gas phase concentrations, which can complicate inter-compound comparisons when markedly dissimilar partition coefficients are involved - Smith and Hall, 1984). In addition, binding of another antagonist cis-2-butene (Sisler and Yang, 1984b) could not be detected in the former system (Bengochea et al., 1980b), whereas in mung bean preparations binding was readily apparent, with an affinity (K_d ca. 10^{-6}M) very much greater than that of the physiologically inactive trans isomer. As discussed in Chapter 1.2., it was suggested that such antagonists act by occupying the binding site without effecting a conformational change.

In many other respects the mung bean cell-free system (references cited) resembles that from French bean - in terms of its ethylene affinity (Table 6.4), particulate nature (maximum activity in the 12,000g-100,000g fraction) lipophilicity, solubilisation by Triton X-100, and inhibition both by thiol reagents (e.g. p-mercuribenzoate) and by thiols - perhaps suggesting the involvement of both a cysteine residue and a disulphide linkage at the binding site. However, the binding activity in mung bean extracts could be precipitated at pH 4 or with ammonium sulphate (or with acetone) and fractionated on a cation exchange column, permitting extensive purification (Table 6.5) by a combination of conventional procedures. In addition to

Table 6.5 - Purification of ethylene-binding component from mung bean sprouts (Sisler, 1980)

Fraction	Total binding dpm/g tissue	Specific activity dpm/mg protein
Crude extract	102.7	6.85
pH 4 precipitate	79.1	7.19
Triton X-100 extract	91.5	183
CM-Sephadex eluate	54.4	1089

thiol compounds, the effects of a wide range of reagents on binding were examined in mung bean extracts. Of particular interest, in relation to the

142

suggested involvement of Cu^+ in ethylene binding at the receptor site (see Chapter 1.2.), is the observed inhibition by thiourea and diethyl-dithiocarbamate, as well as by o-phenanthroline (Table 6.6). In addition, Ag^+ ions, known to antagonise ethylene action, are also potent inhibitors of binding - though in particulate preparations from French bean (Bengochea et al., 1980a), no inhibition by Ag^+ was seen even at 100 mM. Another finding of interest (Table 6.6) was inhibition by KI (but not KCl), an observation that might be related to the ethylene-like response produced by KI on bean abscission (Herrett et al., 1962).

Table 6.6 - Inhibition of ethylene-^{14}C binding to a Triton X-100 extract from mung beans (Sisler, 1982a)

Compound	Concentration (mM)	% inhibition
Thiourea	1	56
Diethyldithiocarbamate	1	54
o-Phenanthroline	1	66
o-Phenanthroline	10	90
$AgNO_3$	0.01	62
$AgNO_3$	0.1	95
$Ag_2S_2O_3$	0.1	47
$Ag_2S_2O_3$	0.5	65
KI	1	50
KI	10	100
KCl	200	0

Can these various ethylene-binding sites be considered as receptors? Their general affinity and selectivity properties and the effect of Ag^+ (in mung bean extracts) would be compatible with such a role. In carnations the K_d for ethylene matches the half-maximal concentration for acceleration of flower senescence, and $Ag_2S_2O_3$ and 2,5-norbornadiene, both of which delay flower senescence, also inhibit ethylene binding in petals (Sisler et al., 1985). In tobacco leaves there is good agreement between the K_d values for ethylene, propene and carbon monoxide, and the half-maximal concentrations for stimulation of respiration in the same tissue (Sisler, 1979). However, CO_2, a competitive inhibitor of ethylene action (K_i 1.55% in the gas phase, Burg and Burg, 1967), is completely without effect (at 10%) on ethylene binding to mung bean extracts (Sisler, 1982a). In French bean, CO_2 inhibits binding in particulate cotyledon preparations (Bengochea et al., 1980b), but stimulates in solubilised extracts (Thomas et al., 1984). Further, there is no known physiological response of bean cotyledons to ethylene (which is not to say that the tissue is necessarily non-responsive, cf. Chapter 1.4.), and the very slow rates of association and dissociation are difficult to reconcile with a receptor role. On the other hand, the techniques used would only detect binding sites with slow rates of dissociation. Work in progress is directed towards purification of the Phaseolus ethylene-binding protein(s) for immunisation purposes in the hope that the antibodies produced can be used to probe for rapidly-dissociating sites with kinetic characteristics more in keeping with those of a receptor, and for binding sites that may be present in responsive tissues (e.g. abscission zones) at much lower concentrations (Smith and Hall, 1985). In tomatoes very little difference was found between normal plants and non-ripening mutants nor and rin in terms of ethylene binding affinity or site concentration in either fruit or leaves (Sisler, 1982b). If, therefore, the binding sites are receptors, it must be concluded that failure to ripen is not a consequence of defective binding of ethylene to its receptors. Mutant receptors might be able to bind ethylene, but have some lesion in response coupling - or the binding sites may just not be receptors.

Finally, mention should be made of the extensive investigations by Beyer and by Hall and co-workers on ethylene oxidation, carried out initially with Pisum sativum and with Vicia faba respectively (see reviews by Dodds and Hall, 1982; Smith and Hall, 1984). In Vicia, ethylene oxide is the sole primary product, whereas in Pisum both CO_2 and ethylene oxide are formed, the latter being normally found as ethylene glycol and its glucose conjugate (Blomstrom and Beyer, 1980) and referred to as 'tissue incorporation'. Cell-free preparations from Vicia were obtained that catalysed the oxidation of ethylene to ethylene oxide with high affinity (Dodds et al., 1979) and subsequently rates comparable to those seen in vivo were obtained in NADPH-dependent microsomal preparations (Smith et al., 1985). Beyer has proposed that ethylene metabolism is an integral part of the mechanism of action of ethylene, i.e. that oxidation is the price that ethylene pays in order to exert its action. This thesis is based on several lines of evidence (summarised in Beyer, 1981), e.g. correlations between acquisition of ethylene sensitivity and onset of oxidation activity, and between inhibition of ethylene action and of metabolism (Fig. 6.12). It is also intriguing that

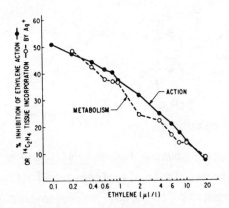

Fig. 6.12 - Inhibition of ethylene action (growth inhibition) and ethylene metabolism in pea seedlings (Beyer, 1979)

ethylene oxide can apparently synergise ethylene action in pea seedlings (Beyer, 1981). Arising from such observations and from similarities in relative affinities for ethylene and analogues, it has been suggested that binding and oxidation activities may represent different manifestations of a common system involved in the regulation of a plant's response to ethylene (Smith and Hall, 1984). Immunochemical approaches should help to throw light on such possible relationships. It is worth noting that in tobacco leaves, ethylene binding was doubled under a nitrogen atmosphere in the presence of $CrCl_2$ as an oxygen scavenger (Goren and Sisler, 1984). Evidently if ethylene oxidation is necessary for ethylene action, binding does not itself require oxygen. During attempted oxidation of ethylene by mammalian cytochrome P-450 monooxygenase, the prosthetic heme forms an hydroxyethyl adduct, thereby undergoing suicide inactivation (Oritz de Montellano et al., 1981). A similar process has not yet been shown in plants, but the Vicia enzyme appears to be a monooxygenase (Smith et al., 1985) and it is intriguing to speculate that such a suicide mechanism might be related to some aspects of ethylene action.

6.5. FUSICOCCIN

Fusicoccin

Fusicoccin is a phytotoxin produced by the fungus Fusicoccum amygdali, a pathogen on peach and almond trees. It is also formed in host tissues infected by the fungus, but otherwise is normally foreign to plants. Despite its very restricted natural distribution, fusicoccin is of considerable physiological interest because of its ability to evoke very rapidly, and at low concentration, certain characteristically hormonal responses in plants, notably H^+ extrusion, K^+ uptake, membrane hyperpolarization, stomatal opening and cell enlargement (Marré, 1979). It is thought that both the pathological and physiological effects of fusicoccin derive from activation of a H^+/K^+ exchange system driven by a plasma membrane ATPase. Because fusicoccin acts more rapidly than auxins for example, it may activate the putative ATPase more directly, and different sets of ATPases may be involved (Marré, 1979; Stout and Cleland, 1980; Cleland, 1982; Hanson and Trewavas, 1982).

A specific and plasma membrane-related action of fusicoccin is supported by the occurrence of high affinity binding sites for the toxin in microsomal preparations of all tissues that have been examined. For these studies, tritiated dihydrofusicoccin (FC-^{3}H) has been used since it can be prepared at high specific activity by catalytic tritiation of the fusicoccin t-pentenyl residue. Fortunately, fusicoccin and its dihydro analogue have essentially identical biological activities (Aducci et al., 1982b). Fusicoccin binding was first detected in membranes from maize coleoptiles (Dohrmann et al., 1977) and has been most extensively studied in this and

146

other tissues of maize and also in spinach leaves (Table 6.7). Binding affinites are high and the concentrations of binding sites are low.

Table 6.7 - Kinetic properties of FC-^{3}H binding sites (membrane-bound except as noted)

Tissue	K_d nM	n pmol/g tissue	Reference
Maize coleoptiles	2	0.7	Dohrmann et al., 1977
Maize coleoptiles	1.2	2.4	Pesci et al., 1979a
	19*	1.2*	
Maize coleoptiles	0.7	0.17	Ballio et al., 1980
	6	0.40[/]	
Maize coleoptiles	0.33	N.R.	Aducci et al., 1984a
	13	N.R.	
Maize leaves	3[‡]	N.R.	Radice et al., 1981
Maize roots	0.9	N.R.	Aducci et al., 1982b
	10	N.R.	
Spinach leaves	5.7	1.4	Ballio et al., 1980
	22	2.6[/]	
Spinach leaves	0.8	0.10*	Aducci et al., 1982a
(solubilized sites)	14	0.56*	

* Values interpolated from the published Scatchard plots

[/] Published n_2 values are actually $n_1 + n_2$ and have been approximately corrected by subtraction of apparent n_1 values

[‡] Approximate 50% displacement value (see data in Fig. 6.13)

N.R. = not reported

147

Scatchard plots, where presented, are normally biphasic and have been interpreted in terms of two sets of binding sites. A two-site model also gave the best fit to the data when dissociation constants were derived with a non-linear least squares fitting programme (Aducci et al., 1984a). Site concentrations were not given, because the analysis used was relatively insensitive to variation in the $n_1:n_2$ ratio, such that in different experiments the apparent proportion of higher affinity sites varied from 1-10% of the total. The Scatchard analyses yield far less unequal n_1 and n_2 values, though in all cases these were derived from direct intercepts and will diverge somewhat after correction (Hunston, 1975). If the true ratio does lie in the range suggested by the analyses of Aducci et al. (1984a) and if only the higher affinity sites turn out to be of interest, then their isolation is likely to continue to prove extremely difficult, in spite of recent advances, discussed below.

Fusicoccin binding is a slow, temperature-dependent process, requiring incubation for 1-2 hours at $26^{o}C$ (Dohrmann et al., 1977; Pesci et al., 1979a). On isopycnic centrifugation, binding activity coincided closely with the NPA binding peak, suggesting that the fusicoccin sites are located in the plasma membrane. The high affinity and slow reversibility of fusicoccin binding also enabled such experiments to be carried out after FC-^{3}H labelling of maize coleoptile sections (Beffagna et al., 1979) or crude membrane fractions (Pesci et al., 1979a), with similar results. In oat roots, fusicoccin binding also appeared to be associated with plasma membrane and was largely abolished by elevated temperatures or by trypsin; the trypsin effect was substantially reduced by co-incubation with trypsin inhibitor (Stout and Cleland, 1980). These findings reinforced earlier indications (Pesci et al., 1979a - sensitivity to mercurials, glutaraldehyde and to pH values removed from pH 5.5) that fusicoccin binds to protein components of the membrane. A surface membrane localisation of fusicoccin binding sites is supported by two further pieces of evidence. Firstly, when oat leaf sections are rehydrated after osmotic shock, fusicoccin-stimulated H^+ excretion is reduced, proteins are released to the rehydration medium, and this protein fraction contains saturable fusicoccin binding activity (Rubinstein, 1982). The shock protein appeared to derive predominantly from the cell surface. The other piece of evidence comes from a short report that after brief exposure to a non-permanent fusicoccin conjugate, tobacco leaf protoplasts rapidly agglutinated when treated with anti-fusicoccin antibodies (Aducci et al., 1980). One recent anomalous finding arises from a preliminary autoradiographic study, which indicates a heterodisperse cellular distribution for FC-^{3}H binding (Aducci et al., 1985). Whether this reflects some technical artefact, or true binding to endogenous membranes as well as to the plasma membrane, or whether it might indicate receptor internalization is not yet clear.

Comparison of the biological activities of a wide range of fusicoccin derivatives (Ballio et al., 1981a) with their ability to compete with FC-^{3}H for binding to maize membranes (Ballio et al., 1981b) supports the supposition that the binding sites are receptors that mediate the physiological action of fusicoccin. Although the value of the comparison is limited by the fact that the in vivo biological data were all obtained at physiologically saturating concentrations, nevertheless, the representative examples selected for Table 6.8 illustrate the general correlation. A rather better comparison, albeit confined to two components, is provided by the data of Radice et al. (1981), comparing biological and binding activities of fusicoccin (FC) and its dideacetyl derivative (DAF), both activities being measured in the same tissue, maize leaves (Fig. 6.13). Fusicoccin was several times more active in promoting H$^+$ extrusion from leaf discs and this was paralleled by its greater binding affinity, as reflected in the displacement curves of FC-^{3}H binding.

Fusicoccin receptors or receptor-FC-^{3}H complexes have been solubilized by a variety of methods and from different tissues - by perchlorate (Pesci et al., 1979b; maize coleoptiles), by Triton X-100 (Stout and Cleland, 1980; oat roots) and by the acetone method used for auxin receptors (Aducci et al., 1982a; spinach leaves). In all cases a molecular weight of about 80,000 daltons was obtained, providing further support for the view that the same fusicoccin-binding protein is common to the plasma membrane of all plants. K$^+$-ATPase is solubilized together with fusicoccin-binding protein, but the two activities can be partially resolved by gel filtration of either detergent extracts (Stout and Cleland, 1980) or perchlorate extracts (Tognoli et al., 1979). In the latter case it was also shown that the activities could be completely resolved by disc electrophoresis on non-denaturing gels. Clearly, then, fusicoccin does not bind to the catalytic unit of the ATPase itself. Nevertheless, from the similar inhibitor

Table 6.8 - Comparison of physiological activities of some fusicoccin analogues with their ability to compete for FC-^{3}H binding to maize coleoptile membranes. Growth data were obtained at 10 mg l^{-1}, are means of activities on pea internode and squash cotyledon growth and are expressed relative to fusicoccin = 100 (Ballio et al., 1981a). C_{50} values are the concentrations giving 50% displacement of FC-^{3}H binding. NC = no displacement at 5x10^{-6}M (Ballio et al., 1981b)

Compound	Growth activity	C_{50} nM
Fusicoccin (FC)	100	3.6
Dihydro-FC	114	3.6
Dideacetyl-FC	102	6.0
9-Epidideacetyl-FC	0	NC
Aglycone of FC	43	800
Aglycone of 9-epi-FC	0	NC
Cotylenin A	86	2.8

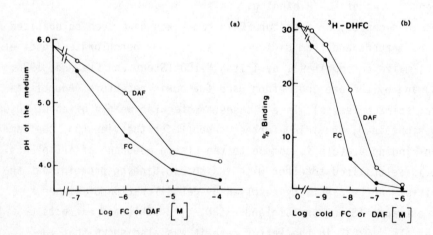

Fig. 6.13 - Effect of FC (●) and DAF (o) on (a) H$^+$ extrusion in maize leaf discs, (b) binding of dihydrofusicoccin-^{3}H by maize leaf membrane preparations (Radice et al., 1981)

sensitivity of the two activities in membrane preparations, it was suggested that they are normally integrated in the membrane in some form of interactive multi-unit complex. Fusicoccin has been reported to stimulate K^+-ATPase in vitro by up to 30% in preparations from both maize coleoptiles and from spinach leaves (Beffagna et al., 1977), but Stout and Cleland (1980) could find no such effect. In view of the experience with auxin, where it appears that the effect is on the K_m for ATP (see Chapter 3.3.), a re-examination at low ATP concentrations may be worthwhile, though the effects reported by Beffagna et al. (1977) were obtained at quite a high ATP concentration (1 mM).

From a variety of methods evaluated, perchlorate solubilization was chosen by Pesci et al. (1979b) because it yielded a single discrete peak of fusicoccin binding on both gel filtration and gel electrophoresis. For preparation of native receptor, other means are needed, however. Stout and Cleland (1980) successfully used Triton X-100, but apart from running the extract on a gel filtration column made no attempt at receptor purification. However, Aducci et al. (1982a) found that the acetone method developed for auxin receptors (Venis, 1977a) was also effective in solubilising the fusicoccin sites (from spinach leaves), the advantage being that the material is obtained in buffer-soluble form, free of detergents or chaotropic agents. It was claimed that the solubilization was nearly quantitative, though this is difficult to reconcile with the apparent site concentrations in the membrane-bound and solubilized states (Table 6.7). Although the apparent K_d for the higher affinity site was also greatly lowered, calculation suggests that the actual total measured FC-^{3}H binding in the solubilized preparations would have been about 40% of that in the membrane preparations. Nevertheless, even this figure represents useful recovery, and obtaining the receptor in buffer-soluble form is an important advance for purification purposes. Efforts in this direction have been hindered by problems of receptor instability, which now appear to have been traced to the action of acid phosphatase and α- mannosidase, both of which were detected in the solubilized preparations (Aducci et al., 1984b). Further addition of commercial samples of these enzymes led to rapid loss of FC-^{3}H binding activity and release of FC-^{3}H already bound (Fig. 6.14); simultaneous addition of both enzymes was more effective than either on its own. Activity of receptor preparations could be effectively stabilized by

addition of 25 mM KF as a phosphatase inhibitor, though the α-mannosidase
inhibitor swainsonine had little effect. It seems therefore that the

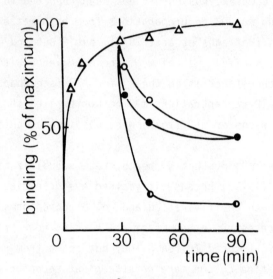

Fig. 6.14 - Binding of FC-^{3}H by spinach leaf solubilised microsomal
preparations. At the arrow, aliquots of mannosidase (o) or acid
phosphatase (●) or both enzymes (◐) were added (Aducci et al., 1984b)

fusicoccin receptor may be a phosphorylated glycoprotein, raising the
possibility that as with certain animal hormone receptors, receptor activity
may be controlled by a phosphorylation-dephosphorylation mechanism (see
Chapter 3.4.) and perhaps by reversible glycosylation also. Now that a means
of improving receptor stability has been found, purification and
investigation of these possibilities should be feasible.

What then is the function of the fusicoccin receptor? In the normal
course of events, cells of most plant species would not expect to encounter
fusicoccin and the binding sites are unlikely to have evolved as a means of
cellular suicide anyway. The logical presumption, as with the NPA receptor,
and following mammalian precedents, is that the fusicoccin receptor normally
binds an as yet unidentified endogenous ligand. Evidence for the existence
of such a ligand was presented by Aducci et al. (1980), who found that FC-^{3}H
binding by maize root membranes was greatly increased (1.3-5.6-fold in
different experiments) if the roots were washed in water for 2 hours prior
to homogenization (Fig. 6.15). Furthermore, if freeze-dried wash was added

to an assay with membranes from either fresh or washed tissue, binding was strongly inhibited, and the wash material also inhibited fusicoccin-

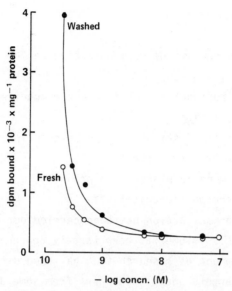

Fig. 6.15 - Displacement by unlabelled fusicoccin of FC-^{3}H binding to microsomal preparations from fresh (o) or washed (•) maize roots (Aducci et al., 1980)

stimulated H$^+$ extrusion from root sections. It was therefore suggested that washing releases an endogenous fusicoccin-like regulator, a suggestion made also by Gronewald et al. (1979) from observations on washing-induced stimulation of H$^+$ extrusion and membrane hyperpolarization. The postulated regulator is considered to have a role in controlling the activity of the H$^+$/K$^+$ exchange system. Presumably fusicoccin removes this control by displacing the ligand from its binding site, or bypassing the normal regulatory mechanism in some way. Hanson and Trewavas (1982) have suggested that the H$^+$/K$^+$ ATPase may be regulated by cytoplasmic Ca^{2+}, but it seems unlikely that the putative endogenous ligand is simply Ca^{2+}. Nevertheless, it would be helpful to know more about some of the basic properties of the inhibitory root wash material, e.g. molecular size, heat and ashing stability and whether its interaction is competitive with fusicoccin. Unfortunately, no further characterization of the wash substance has appeared since the original report in 1980.

7 Summary and Future Prospects

Investigations on the mechanisms of hormone action can be carried out at
several different levels, e.g:-
1. the way in which the hormonal signal is first recognised, i.e. the nature
of hormone-receptor interaction;
2. the nature and mechanism of stimulus-response coupling;
3. identification of the primary response;
4. identification of hormone-regulated gene products;
5. characterisation of end physiological effects.

Most work on plant hormone action has been carried out at levels 4 and 5,
particularly level 5. This volume has been largely concerned with the
relatively very small amount of research that has been directed at level 1.
Levels 2 and 3 remain largely unexplored apart from some direct, and rather
more indirect, evidence that altered ion fluxes (H^+, K^+, Ca^{2+}) are close to
the primary action of at least some hormones, and that in addition
(consequentially or independently) hormones can selectively regulate gene
transcription. Concentration of effort at level 5 has led to a preoccupation
with multiple effects of individual hormones, with the ability of different
hormones to produce somewhat similar end-effects in some circumstances, and
most of all with a bewildering array of interactive effects of different
hormones. Much of this effort has obscured rather than illuminated primary
hormone action. There are many ways in which multiple phenomena can arise
some way downstream from a single primary action, and the existence of
'constant' and 'variable' regions on receptors (cf. antibodies) would be one
means whereby different hormones could trigger similar molecular events
(Strosberg, 1984). However, until very much more attention is paid to levels
1-3, such possibilities - and others, such as response regulation by
receptor internalisation - must remain no more than idle speculation.

Recombinant DNA technology has now established the veracity of the main
premise of much plant hormone work in the 1960s, namely that hormones can
regulate gene transcription - though the identity of the hormone-regulated
genes and the way in which their activity is regulated remains, for the most

part, to be established (Chapter 1.3.). Sequencing of cDNA clones, deduction of amino acid sequence and matching of cDNA and/or polypeptide sequences against libraries, should lead to the identification of some of the gene products. Other (lengthier) approaches to gene function might include Agrobacterium-mediated insertion of cloned hormone-regulated genes modified by site-directed mutagenesis or of genes constructed so as to be transcribed backwards. In the latter case, 'anti-sense' RNA complementary to the normal gene's mRNA will be produced and thereby inhibit its translation by RNA-RNA hybridization. An alternative approach, avoiding the difficult problems of appropriate plasmid construction and gene expression, would be to micro-inject anti-sense RNA into cells or protoplasts (Melton, 1985) and examine the consequences for expression of hormone-mediated responses. Sequencing of hormone-related genomic DNAs should identify consensus upstream sequences which would constitute the sites of presumed interaction with the hormone-receptor complex.

Affinity chromatography and affinity labelling methods have had far less influence in the plant field than they have had with animal hormone receptors. However, ABA receptors have been successfully detected for the first time by means of photoaffinity labelling (Hornberg and Weiler, 1984) and this notable success may stimulate wider interest in the possibilities of affinity labelling techniques. Although the arrival of more efficient column chromatographic procedures for protein fractionation diminishes to some extent the inherent attractions of affinity chromatography, effective hormone affinity adsorbents could still find a place in receptor isolation, particularly in cases where binding is undetectable in crude extracts, e.g. by virtue of low receptor abundance. Experience to date suggests that this approach will only be productive if the utility of the adsorbent has first been validated with fractions from other sources that do contain detectable hormone binding activity - and this may represent Catch 22 in some cases. Receptor reconstitution in bilayer lipid membranes or in liposomes, together with a putative effector, offers possibilities for evaluation of receptor function in a simplified system, but in plants has so far only been attempted in one case (Thompson, M. et al., 1983). Another approach would be to see if hormone responsiveness could be conferred on non-target cells by fusion of protoplasts with liposomes containing inserted receptors (Cerione et al., 1983) or even by direct receptor-protoplast incorporation. Improved methods for isolation and fractionation of cellular membranes from plant tissues would help to resolve questions of receptor localisation and provide better-defined fractions than those currently used. One possibility might be selective membrane agglutination using monoclonal antibodies directed against antigens specific to particular membranes, e.g. plasma membrane ATPase (Chin, 1982).

Mutants have scarcely been used at all to evaluate function of hormone binding sites in plants. Several mutants with reduced sensitivity to various hormones have been described, e.g. to ABA in maize (Robichaud et al., 1980), Arabidopsis (Koornneef et al., 1984), tobacco cultures (Wong and Sussex, 1980) and barley (Ho et al., 1980); to GA in certain dwarf wheats (Ho et al., 1981) and in barley (Ho et al., 1980); to cytokinins and to auxin in the moss Physcomitrella (Ashton et al., 1979), and to auxins in Arabidopsis (Maher and Martindale, 1980). Whilst reduced hormone sensitivity could arise for several reasons, in many of the above cases the evidence suggests that the mutation is receptor-related. Even more attractive than mutants in some respects are the possibilities that seem to exist with cereal aleurones for experimental manipulation of sensitivity to gibberellin (Armstrong et al., 1982; Singh and Paleg, 1984). To exploit any of these systems however, the first hurdle that must be overcome is detection of hormone binding in the 'normal' tissue. Thus Lomax-Reichert et al. (1982) were interested in using auxin-insensitive Physcomitrella mutants, but auxin binding in the wild type was barely detectable, and even then only after sucrose gradient fraction-ation of the total membrane preparations. Auxin-resistant Arabidopsis mutants are currently being explored (C. Bell, personal communication), and while initial results are more encouraging than those with Physcomitrella, nevertheless the levels of binding obtained in the wild type are still very low. Perhaps mutants with enhanced rather than attenuated hormone sensitivity should be sought. Alternatively, mutant maize lines could be explored for putative auxin receptor mutants, given that in coleoptile membranes auxin binding is readily detectable and well-characterised; dwarf maize mutants have, of course, proved of great value in elucidating the pathway of gibberellin biosynthesis in this species (Phinney and Spray, 1982).

The current overall position with regard to putative receptor systems for plant hormones and allied regulators can be summarised as follows:-

1. Specific, high affinity binding sites for synthetic auxin transport inhibitors (phytotropins, e.g. NPA) and for fusicoccin can be readily detected in various species. The precise function of these sites remains to be resolved, but their further investigation should contribute to an improved understanding of the mechanisms of auxin transport and auxin action. Since neither phytotropins nor fusicoccin are normally found in plants, it is reasonable to presume, from mammalian precedents, that these receptors usually recognise as yet unknown natural ligands, whose identification could be of both physiological and agrochemical interest.
2. Auxin-binding sites with many properties suggestive of a receptor function have been well characterised in coleoptile membranes of maize and to a much lesser extent in other monocotyledons. Convincing auxin binding in dicotyledonous shoot tissues has yet to be demonstrated. Soluble auxin binding sites have been best studied in tobacco cultures and there is preliminary evidence to suggest that their activity (and that of fusicoccin sites) may be regulated by phosphorylation.
3. Many cytokinin-binding and gibberellin-binding systems have been described, but in no case is there compelling evidence that the binding being studied is to a physiological receptor.
4. ABA receptors have been detected by photoaffinity labelling, and it can be expected that isolation of binding fractions will follow.
5. Ethylene binding sites with appropriate affinities and specificities, but having very slow rates of association and dissociation, have been reported from several sources. It is too early to judge whether or not these represent receptors, but the evidence is sufficiently encouraging to warrant further investigation.

The techniques that are likely to make most impact on plant hormone receptor research in the immediate future are immunochemical ones, particularly the exploitation of monoclonal antibody technology. This has already been successfully applied to localisation of putative auxin efflux carriers (NPA receptors) using monoclonal antibodies raised against crude membrane preparations, and there is no reason why antibodies to other membrane-bound receptors should not be obtained similarly, and even simultaneously - i.e. ABA, fusicoccin and auxin receptors. Indeed, only the absence of suitable screens would prevent such monoclonal populations being searched for antibodies against possible membrane-bound gibberellin and cytokinin receptors. A preliminary report has appeared on a monospecific auxin receptor antibody derived from a polyclonal antiserum, albeit by a somewhat tortuous route. Since maize auxin receptors can be obtained in 10-15% purity with ease, the production of families of monoclonal antibodies should be relatively straightforward.

There is even a possible immunological way forward in those cases where no convincing receptor-containing fractions are available for immunization - i.e. for gibberellins and cytokinins. This approach would make use of the auto-anti-idiotypic response of the immune system, whereby injection of an antigen elicits, in addition to antibodies to the antigen, other antibodies (anti-idiotypic) directed at the antigen-combining sites of the first set. Assuming that macromolecules of the same specificity will show structural homologies in their binding sites, then if the antigen-specific antibodies recognise a hormone, it follows that among the population of anti-idiotypic antibodies there should be some that are in effect hormone receptor antibodies. The success of this approach has been demonstrated, for example in the case of acetylcholine receptors (Cleveland et al., 1983). The strategy, therefore, would be to raise monoclonals against the hormone (e.g. a cytokinin) and then use one or more appropriate antibodies (showing good cross-reactivity between active cytokinins, and suitable selectivity against inactive analogues) to rescreen the 'inactive' hybridoma clones for anti-idiotypic antibodies, by inhibition of cytokinin-cytokinin antibody binding. Among these anti-antibodies one would hope to find some with recognition properties equivalent to those of anti-receptor antibodies. These would need to be selected in some way, e.g. by ability to block a cytokinin-dependent response, or by patterns of immuno-histochemical labelling. They could then be used in immunoaffinity columns for receptor isolation.

This approach would be a circuitous one, with no guarantee of success, but nevertheless worth exploring should other avenues continue to be unproductive. At worst, the investigator would end up with a supply of monoclonal antibodies to the hormone. Alternatively, since hormone monoclonals have been and are being produced in several laboratories, and are also available commercially, it may be possible to shorten the procedure by immunizing instead with the hormone antibodies - though the criteria used to select the monoclonal for hormone assay purposes may not necessarily be the most favourable for generation of anti-receptor antibodies.

The total effort devoted to investigation of plant receptors is only a very small proportion of that applied to animal receptor studies - probably less than 1% - so it is not surprising that the levels of understanding are very different. There are, nevertheless, indications of accelerating progress with plant hormone receptors and the next decade could be a fruitful and exciting period. Every encouragement should be given to those seeking to enter this field and thereby contribute to the elucidation of plant hormone action at the molecular level.

References

Abe, H., Morishita, T., Uchiyama, M., Takatsuto, S., Ikekawa, N., Ikeda, M., Sassa, T., Kitsuwa, T., and Marumo, S. (1983). Occurrence of three brassinosteroids: brassinone, (24S)-24-ethylbrassinone and 28-norbrassinolide, in higher plants. Experientia 39, 351-353.

Abe, H., Morishita, T., Uchiyama, M., Takatsuto, S. and Ikekawa, N. (1984). A new brassinolide-related steroid in the leaves of Thea sinensis. Agric. Biol. Chem. 48, 2171-2172.

Abeles, F.B. (1973). Ethylene in Plant Biology. Academic Press, London.

Aducci, P., Federico, R. and Ballio, A. (1980). Fusicoccin receptors. Evidence for an endogenous ligand. Planta 148, 208-210.

Aducci, P., Ballio, A. and Federico, R. (1982a). Solubilisation of fusicoccin binding sites. In: 'Plasmalemma and Tonoplast. Their Function in the Plant Cell'. (D. Marmé, F. Marrè and R. Hertel, eds.). pp 279-284. Elsevier Biomedical Press, Amsterdam.

Aducci, P., Ballio, A., Federico, R. and Montesano, L. (1982b). Studies on fusicoccin-binding sites. In: 'Plant Growth Substances 1982'. (P.F. Wareing, ed.). pp 395-404. Academic Press, London - New York.

Aducci, P., Coletta, M. and Marra, M. (1984a). An improved Scatchard analysis of fusicoccin-binding to maize coleoptile membranes. Plant Sci. Lett. 33, 187-193.

Aducci, P., Ballio, A., Fiorucci, L. and Simonetti, E. (1984b). Inactivation of solubilised fusicoccin-binding sites by endogenous plant hydrolases. Planta 160, 422-427.

Aducci, P., Ballio, A. and Autuori, F. (1985). Fusicoccin binding sites: an autoradiographic study. Phytopath. med. (in press).

Amrhein, N. (1977). The current status of cyclic AMP in plants. Ann. Rev. Plant Physiol. 28, 123-132.

Armstrong, C., Black, M., Chapman, J.M., Norman, H.A. and Angold, R. (1982). The induction of sensitivity to gibberellin in aleurone tissue of developing wheat grains. I. The effect of dehydration. Planta 154, 573-577.

Ashton, N.W., Grimsley, N.H. and Cove, D.J. (1979). Analysis of gametophytic development in the moss, Physcomitrella patens using auxin and cytokinin resistant mutants. Planta 144, 427-435.

Atkins, G.L. and Nimmo, I.A. (1975). A comparison of seven methods of fitting the Michaelis-Menton equation. Biochem. J. 149, 775-777.

Audus, L.J. (1972). Plant Growth Substances, Vol. I. Leonard Hill, London.

Auricchio, F., Migliaccio, A., Castoria, G., Rotondi, A. and Lastoria, S. (1984). Direct evidence of in vitro phosphorylation of the estradiol-17β-receptor. Role of Ca^{2+}-calmodulin in the activation of hormone binding sites. J. Steroid Biochem. 20, 31-35.

Bagni, N., Fracassini, S. and Torrigiani, P. (1982). Polyamines and cellular growth processes in higher plants. In: 'Plant Growth Substances 1982'. (P.F. Wareing, ed.). pp 473-482. Academic Press, London - New York.

Ballio, A., Federico, R., Pessi, A. and Scalorbi, D. (1980). Fusicoccin binding sites in subcellular preparations of spinach leaves. Plant Sci. Lett. 18, 39-44.

Ballio, A., De Michelis, M.I., Lado, P. and Randazzo, G. (1981a). Fusicoccin structure-activity relationships: Stimulation of growth by cell enlargement and promotion of seed germination. Physiol. Plant. 52, 471-475.

Ballio, A., Federico, R. and Scalorbi, D. (1981b). Fusicoccin structure-activity relationships. In vitro binding to microsomal preparations of maize coleoptiles. Physiol. Plant. 52, 476-481.

Batt, S. and Venis, M.A. (1976). Separation and localization of two classes of auxin binding sites in corn coleoptile membranes. Planta 130, 15-21.

Batt, S., Wilkins, M.B. and Venis, M.A. (1976). Auxin binding to corn coleoptile membranes: kinetics and specificity. Planta 130, 7-13.

Bayley, H. and Knowles, J.R. (1977). Photoaffinity labelling. Methods in Enzymology 46, 69-114.

Bearder, J.R. (1980). Plant hormones and other growth substances. Their background, structures and occurrence. In: 'Hormonal Regulation of Development'. Encyclopedia of Plant Physiology, New Series Vol. 9. (J. MacMillan, ed.). pp 9-112. Springer-Verlag, Berlin - Heidelberg - New York.

Beffagna, N., Cocucci, S. and Marrè, E. (1977). Stimulating effect of fusicoccin on K-activated ATPase in plasmalemma preparations from higher plant tissues. Plant Sci. Lett. 8, 91-98.

Beffagna, N., Pesci. P., Tognoli, L. and Marrè, E. (1979). Distribution of fusicoccin bound in vivo among subcellular fractions from maize coleoptiles. Plant Sci. Lett. 15, 323-330.

Beggs, M.J. and Sisler, E.C. (1985). Binding of ethylene analogs and cyclic olefins to a Triton X-100 extract from plants: Comparison with in vivo activities. Plant Growth Regul. (in press).

Bengochea, T., Dodds, J.H., Evans, D.E., Jerie, P.H., Niepel, B., Shari, A.R. and Hall, M.A. (1980a). Studies on ethylene binding by cell-free preparations from cotyledons of Phaseolus vulgaris L.: Separation and characterisation. Planta 148, 397-406.

Bengochea, T., Acaster, M.A., Dodds, J.H., Evans, D.E., Jerie, P.H. and Hall, M.A. (1980b). Studies on ethylene binding by cell-free preparations from cotyledons of Phaseolus vulgaris L.: Effects of structural analogues of ethylene and of inhibitors. Planta 148, 407-411.

Berridge, M.J. and Irvine, R.E. (1984). Inositol triphosphate, a novel second messenger in cellular signal transduction. Nature (London) 312, 315-321.

Berridge, M.V., Ralph, R.K. and Letham, D.S. (1970). The binding of cytokinin to plant ribosomes. Biochem. J. 119, 75-84.

Beyer, F.M. (1976). A potent inhibitor of ethylene action in plants. Plant Physiol. 58, 268-271.

Beyer, F.M. (1979). Effect of silver ion, carbon dioxide and oxygen on ethylene action and metabolism. Plant Physiol. 63, 169-173.

Beyer, F.M. (1981). Recent advances in ethylene metabolism. In: 'Aspects and Prospects of Plant Growth Regulators'. (B. Jeffcoat, ed.). pp 27-38. Wessex Press, Wantage.

Bhattacharyya, K. and Biswas, B.B. (1982). Induction of a high affinity binding site for auxin in Avena root membrane. Phytochemistry 21, 1207-1211.

Biswas, B.B., Ganguly, A., Das, A. and Roy, P. (1975). Action of indoleacetic acid: a plant growth hormone on transcription. In: 'Regulation of Growth and Differentiated Function in Eukaryote Cells'. (G.P. Talwar, ed.). pp 461-477. Raven Press, New York.

Bittner, S., Gorodetsky, M., Har-Paz, I., Mizrahi, Y. and Richmond, A.E. (1977). Synthesis and biological effects of aromatic analogs of abscisic acid. Phytochemistry 16, 1143-1151.

Blomstrom, D.C. and Beyer, F.M. (1980). Plants metabolise ethylene to ethylene glycol. Nature (London) 283, 66-68.

Boeynaems, J.M. and Dumont, J.E. (1980). Outlines of Receptor Theory. Elsevier Biomedical Press, Amsterdam - New York - Oxford.

Bogers, R.J., Kulescha, Z., Quint, A., Van Vliet, T.B. and Libbenga, K.R. (1980). The presence of a soluble auxin receptor and the metabolism of 3-indoleacetic acid in tobacco-pith explants. Plant Sci. Lett. 19, 311-317.

Bradley, P.M., El-Fiki, F. and Giles, K.L. (1984). Polyamines and arginine affect somatic embryogenesis of Daucus carota. Plant Sci. Lett. 34, 397-401.

Bressan, R.A., Ross, C.W. and Vandepeute, J. (1976). Attempts to detect cyclic adenosine 3':5'-monophosphate in higher plants by three assay methods. Plant Physiol. 57, 29-37.

Brian, P.W., Grove, J.F. and Mulholland, T.P.C. (1967). Relationships between structure and growth-promoting activity of the gibberellins and some allied compounds in four test systems. Phytochemistry 6, 1475-1499.

Briggs, D.E. (1966). Gibberellin-like activity of helminthosporol and helminthosporic acid. Nature (London) 210, 418-419.

Brinegar, A.C. and Fox, J.E. (1985). Resolution of the subunit composition of a cytokinin-binding protein from wheat embryos. Biol. Plantarum (in press).

Brown, E.G. and Newton, R.P. (1981). Cyclic AMP and higher plants. Phytochemistry 20, 2453-2463.

Bruce, M.I. and Zwar, J.A. (1966). Cytokinin activity of some substituted ureas and thioureas. Proc. Roy. Soc. B 165, 245-265.

Buckhout, T.J., Young, K.A., Low, P.S. and Morré, D.J. (1981). In vitro promotion by auxins of divalent cation release from soybean membranes. Plant Physiol. 68, 512-515.

Burg, S.P. and Burg, E.A. (1967). Molecular requirements for the biological activity of ethylene. Plant Physiol. 42, 144-152.

Burrows, W.J. (1978). Cytokinins. Biochem. Soc. Trans. 6, 1395-1400.

Cerione, R.A., Strulovici, B., Benovic, J.L., Lefkowitz, R.J. and Caron, M.G. (1983). Pure β-adrenergic receptor: the single polypeptide confers catecholamine responsiveness to adenylate cyclase. Nature (London) 306, 562-566.

Chapman, K.S.R., Trewavas, A. and Van Loon, L.C. (1975). Regulation of the phosphorylation of chromatin-associated proteins in Lemna and Hordeum. Plant Physiol. 55, 293-296.

Chen, C., Melitz, D.K., Petschow, B. and Eckert, R.L. (1980). Isolation of cytokinin-binding protein from plant tissues by affinity chromatography. Eur. J. Biochem. 108, 379-387.

Cheng, Y. and Prusoff, W.H. (1973). Relationship between the inhibition constant (K_i) and the concentration of inhibitor which causes 50 per cent inhibition (I_{50}) of an enzymatic reaction. Biochem. Pharmacol. 22, 3099-3108.

Cheung, W.Y. (1980). Calmodulin plays a pivotal role in cellular regulation. Science 207, 19-27.

Chin, J.J.C. (1982). Monoclonal antibodies that immunoreact with a cation-stimulated plant membrane ATPase. Biochem. J. 203, 51-54.

Chung, S.R., Durand, R. and Durand, B. (1979). Differential cytokinin binding to dioecious plant ribosomes. FEBS letters 102, 211-215.

Clark, A.J. (1933). Mode of Action of Drugs on Cells. Arnold, London.

Clark, J.E., Morré, D.J., Cherry, J.H. and Yunghans, W.N. (1976). Enhancement of RNA polymerase activity by non-protein components from plasma membranes of soybean hypocotyl. Plant Sci. Lett. 7, 233-238.

Cleland, R. (1973). Auxin-induced hydrogen ion excretion from Avena coleoptiles. Proc. Natl. Acad. Sci. USA 70, 3092-3093.

Cleland, R. (1982). The mechanism of auxin-induced proton efflux. In: 'Plant Growth Substances 1982'. (P.F. Wareing, ed.). pp 23-31. Academic Press, London - New York.

Cleveland, W.L., Wassermann, N.H., Sarangarajan, R., Penn, A.S. and Erlanger, B.F. (1983). Monoclonal antibodies to the acetylcholine receptor by a normally functioning auto-anti-idiotypic mechanism. Nature (London) 305, 56-57.

Cohen, J.D. and Lilly, N. (1984). Changes in ^{45}calcium concentration following auxin treatment of protoplasts isolated from etiolated soybean hypocotyls. Plant Physiol. 75 S, 109.

Colowick, S.P. and Womack, F.C. (1969). Binding of diffusible molecules by macromolecules: rapid measurement by rate of dialysis. J. Biol. Chem. 244, 774-777.

Cross, J.W. and Briggs, W.R. (1978). Properties of a solubilized auxin-binding protein from coleoptiles and primary leaves of Zea mays. Plant Physiol. 62, 152-157.

Cross, J.W., Briggs, W.R., Dohrmann, U.C. and Ray, P.M. (1978). Auxin receptors of maize coleoptile membranes do not have ATPase activity. Plant Physiol. 61, 581-584.

Crozier, A., Kuo, C.C., Durley, R.C. and Pharis, R.P. (1970). The biological activities of 26 gibberellins in nine plant bioassays. Can J. Bot. 48, 867-877.

Cuatrecasas, P., Wilchek, M. and Anfinsen, C.B. (1968). Selective enzyme purification by affinity chromatography. Proc. Natl. Acad. Sci. USA 61, 636-643.

Dai, Y.R., Kaur-Sawkney, R. and Galston, A.W. (1982). Promotion by gibberellic acid of polyamine biosynthesis in internodes of light-grown dwarf peas. Plant Physiol. 69, 103-105.

Davies, E. and Maclachlan, G.A. (1969). Effects of indoleacetic acid on intracellular distribution of β-glucanase activities in the pea epicotyl. Archs. Biochem. Biophys. 129, 581-587.

Depta, H., Eisele, K.-H., and Hertel, R. (1983). Specific inhibitors of auxin transport: action on tissue segments and in vitro binding to membranes from maize coleoptiles. Plant Sci. Lett. 31, 181-192.

Dieter, P. (1984). Calmodulin and calmodulin-mediated processes in plants. Plant Cell Environment 7, 371-380.

Dixon, M. and Webb, E.C. (1958). Enzymes. Longman's, London.

Dodds, J.H. and Hall, M.A. (1982). Metabolism of ethylene by plants. Int. Rev. Cytol. 76, 299-325.

Dodds, J.H., Musa, S.K., Jerie, P.H. and Hall, M.A. (1979). Metabolism of ethylene to ethylene oxide by cell-free preparations from Vicia faba. Plant Sci. Lett. 17, 109-114.

Dohrmann, U., Hertel, R., Pesci. P., Cocucci, S.M., Marre, E., Randazzo, G. and Ballio, A. (1977). Localization of "in vitro" binding of the fungal toxin fusicoccin to plasma-membrane rich fractions from corn coleoptiles. Plant Sci. Lett 9, 291-299.

Dohrmann, U., Hertel, R. and Kowalik, H. (1978). Properties of auxin binding sites in different subcellular fractions from maize coleoptiles. Planta 140, 97-106.

Dollstädt, R., Hirschberg, K., Winkler, E. and Hubner, G. (1976). Bindung von Indolylessigsäure und Phenoxyessigsäure an Fraktionen aus Epikotylen und Wurzeln von Pisum sativum L. Planta 130, 105-111.

Eisenthal, R. and Cornish-Bowden, A. (1974). The direct linear plot. A new graphical procedure for estimating enzyme kinetic parameters. Biochem. J. 139, 715-720.

Elliott, D.C. (1983). Inhibition of cytokinin-regulated responses by calmodulin-binding compounds. Plant Physiol. 72, 215-218.

Elliott, D.C., Batchelor, S.M., Cassar, R.A., and Marinos, N.G. (1983). Calmodulin-binding drugs affect responses to cytokinins, auxin and gibberellic acid. Plant Physiol. 72, 219-224.

Erdei, L., Toth, I. and Zsoldos, F. (1979). Hormonal regulation of Ca^{2+}-stimulated K^+ influx and Ca^{2+}, K^+-ATPase in rice roots: in vivo and in vitro effects of auxins and reconstitution of the ATPase. Physiol. Plant. 45, 448-452.

Erion, J.L. and Fox, J.E. (1981). Purification and properties of a protein which binds cytokinin-active 6-substituted purines. Plant Physiol. 67, 156-162.

Ernst, D., Schäfer, W. and Oesterhelt, D. (1983). Isolation and identification of a new, naturally occurring cytokinin (6-benzyl-aminopurine riboside) from an anise cell culture. Planta 159, 222-225.

Evans, D.E., Bengochea, T., Cairns, A.J., Dodds, J.H. and Hall, M.A. (1982a). Studies on ethylene binding by cell-free preparations from cotyledons of Phaseolus vulgaris L.: subcellular localization. Plant Cell Environment 5, 101-107.

Evans, D.E., Dodds, J.H., Lloyd, P.C., ap Gwynn, I. and Hall, M.A. (1982b). A study of the subcellular localisation of an ethylene binding site in developing cotyledons of Phaseolus vulgaris L. by high resolution autoradiography. Planta 154, 48-52.

Evans, M.L. (1974). Rapid responses of plant hormones. Ann. Rev. Plant. Physiol. 25, 195-224.

Fan, D.F. and Maclachlan, G.A. (1966). Control of cellulase activity by indoleacetic acid. Can. J. Bot. 44, 1025-1034.

Farrimond, J.A., Elliott, M.C. and Clack, D.W. (1978). Charge separation as a component of the structural requirements for hormone activity. Nature (London) 274, 401-402.

Farrimond, J.A., Elliott, M.C. and Clack, D.W. (1980). Auxin structure/activity relationships: benzoic acids and phenols. Phytochemistry 19, 367-371.

Farrimond, J.A., Elliott, M.C., and Clack, D.W. (1981). Auxin structure/activity relationships: aryloxyacetic acids. Phytochemistry 20, 1185-1190.

Feirer, R.P., Mignon, G. and Litvay, J.D. (1984). Arginine decarboxylase and polyamines required for embryogenesis in the wild carot. Science 223, 1433-1435.

Feldmann, H.A. (1972). Mathematical theory of complex ligand-binding systems at equilibrium. Some methods for parameter fitting. Anal. Biochem. 48, 317-338.

Feldmann, K. (1978). New devices for flow dialysis and ultrafiltration for the study of protein-ligand interactions. Anal. Biochem. 88, 225-235.

Firn, R.D. and Digby, J. (1980). The establishment of tropic curvatures in plants. Ann. Rev. Plant Physiol. 31, 131-148.

Firn, R.D. and Kearns, A.W. (1982). The search for the auxin receptor. In: 'Plant Growth Substances 1982'. (P.F. Wareing, ed.). pp 385-393. Academic Press, London - New York.

Fox, J.E. and Erion, J.L. (1975). A cytokinin binding protein from higher plant ribosomes. Biochem. Biophys. Res. Commun. 64, 694-700.

Fox, J.E. and Erion, J.L. (1977). Cytokinin binding proteins in higher plants. In: 'Plant Growth Regulation'. (P.-E. Pilet, ed.). pp 139-146. Springer, Berlin - Heidelberg - New York.

Fox, J.E. and Gregerson, E. (1982). Variation in a cytokinin binding protein among several cereal crop plants. In: 'Plant Growth Substances 1982'. (P.F. Wareing, ed.). pp 207-214. Academic Press, London - New York.

Gabathuler, R. and Cleland, R.F. (1984). Characterization of electrogenic proton uptake, stimulated by nitrate and IAA, into pea root membrane vesicles. Plant Physiol. 75 S, 22.

Gabathuler, R., Moloney, M.M. and Pilet, P.E. (1983). Possible regulation by IAA of an ATP-dependent electrogenic proton uptake into maize and pea root membrane vesicles. Plant Physiol. 72 S, 116.

Galston, A.W. (1983). Polamines as modulators of plant development. BioScience 36, 382-388.

Garcia, T., Tuohimaa, P., Mester, J., Buchon, T., Renoir, J.-M. and Baulieu, E.-E. (1983). Protein kinase activity of purified components of the chicken oviduct progesterone receptor. Biochem. Biophys. Res. Commun. 113, 960-966.

Gardner, G. Sussman, M.R. and Kende, H. (1978). In vitro cytokinin binding to a particulate cell fraction from protonemata of Funaria hygrometrica. Planta 143, 67-73.

Geuns, J.M.C. (1978). Review: Steroid hormones and plant growth and development. Phytochemistry 17, 1-14.

Geuns, J.M.C. (1983). Structural requirements of corticosteroids in etiolated mung bean seedlings. Z. Pflanzenphysiol. 111, 141-154.

Goeldner, M.P., Hirth, C.G., Kieffer, B. and Ourisson, G. (1982). Photosuicide inhibition - a step towards specific photoaffinity labelling. Trends Biochem. Sci. 7, 310-312.

Goren, R. and Sisler, E.L. (1984). Ethylene binding: some parameters in excised tobacco leaves. Tobacco Sci. 62, 110-115.

Goren, R. and Sisler, E.L. (1985). Ethylene-binding characteristics in Phaseolus, Citrus, and Ligustrum plants. Plant Growth Regul. (in press).

Graebe, J.E. and Ropers, H.J. (1978). Gibberellins. In: 'Phytohormones and Related Compounds: A Comprehensive Treatise'. (D.S. Letham, P.B. Goodwin and T.J.V. Higgins, eds.). Vol. 1, pp 107-204. Elsevier Biomedical Press, Amsterdam - Oxford - New York.

Gronemeyer, H. and Pongs, O. (1980). Localization of ecdysterone on polytene chromosomes of Drosophila melanogaster. Proc. Natl. Acad. Sci. USA 77, 2108-2112.

Gronewald, J.W., Cheeseman, J.M. and Hanson. J.B. (1979). Comparison of the responses of corn root tissue to fusicoccin and washing. Plant Physiol. 63, 255-259.

Grove, M.D., Spencer, G.F., Rohwedder, W.K., Mandava, N., Worley, J.F.,
Worthen, J.D., Steffens, G.L., Flippen-Anderson, J.L. and Cook, J.C.
(1979). Brassinolide, a plant growth-promoting steroid isolated from
Brassica napus pollen. Nature (London) 281, 216-217.

Guzman, C.C. de and Fuente, R.K. de la (1984). Polar calcium flux in
sunflower hypocotyl segments. I. The effect of auxin. Plant Physiol.
76, 347-352.

Hagen, G., Kleinschmidt, A. and Guilfoyle, T. (1984). Auxin-regulated gene
expression in intact soybean hypocotyl and excised hypocotyl sections.
Planta 162, 147-153.

Hager, A., Menzel, H. and Krauss, A. (1971). Versuche und Hypothese zur
Primärwirkung des Auxin beim Streckungswachstum. Planta 100, 47-75.

Hall, J.L. (1983). Plasma membranes. In: 'Isolation of Membranes and
Organelles from Plant Cells'. (J.L. Hall and A.L. Moore, eds.). pp 55-
81. Academic Press, London.

Hall, M.A., Smith, A.R., Thomas, C.J.R. and Howarth, C.J. (1984). Binding
sites for ethylene. In: 'Ethylene: Biochemical, Physiological and
Applied Aspects'. (Y. Fuchs and F. Chalutz, eds.). pp 55-63. Martinus
Nijhoff/Dr. W. Junk, The Hague.

Hansch, C., Muir, R.M. and Metzenberg, R.L. (1951). Further evidence for a
chemical reaction between plant growth regulators and a plant substrate.
Plant Physiol. 26, 812-821.

Hanson, J.B. and Trewavas, A.J. (1982). Regulation of plant cell growth:
the changing perspective. New Phytol. 90, 1-18.

Harada, H. (1980). Cytokinin-binding protein in grape berries. Vitis 19,
216-225.

Hardin, J.W. and Cherry, J.G. (1972). Solubilization and partial
characterization of soybean chromatin-bound RNA polymerase. Biochem.
Biophys. Res. Commun. 48, 299-306.

Hardin, J.W., O'Brien, T.J. and Cherry, J.H. (1970). Stimulation of
chromatin bound RNA polymerase activity by a soluble factor. Biochim.
Biophys. Acta 224, 667-670.

Hardin, J.W., Cherry, J.H., Morré, D.J. and Lembi, C.A. (1972). Enhancement
of soybean RNA polymerase activity by a factor released by auxin from
isolated fractions enriched in plasma membranes. Proc. Natl. Acad. Sci.
USA 69, 3146-3150.

Harper, D.B. and Wain, R.L. (1969). Studies on plant growth-regulating
substances. XXX The plant growth-regulating activity of substituted
phenols. Ann. Appl. Biol. 64, 395-407.

Helgerson, S.L., Cramer, W.A. and Morré, D.J. (1976). Evidence for an increase in microviscosity of plasma membranes from soybean hypocotyls induced by the plant hormone, indole-3-acetic acid. Plant Physiol. 58, 548-551.

Herrett, R.A., Hatfield, H.H., Crosby, D.G. and Vlitos, A.J. (1962). Leaf abscission induced by the iodide ion. Plant Physiol. 37, 358-363.

Hertel, R. (1974). Auxin transport and in vitro auxin binding. In: 'Membrane Transport in Plants'. (U. Zimmermann and J. Dainty, eds.). pp 457-461. Springer, Berlin - Heidelberg - New York.

Hertel, R. (1983). The mechanism of auxin transport as a model for auxin action. Z. Pflanzenphysiol. 112, 53-67.

Hertel, R., Thomson, K-St., and Russo, V.E.A. (1972). In vitro auxin binding to particulate cell fractions from corn coleoptiles. Planta 107, 325-340.

Hertel, R., Dohrmann, U., Jesaitis, A.J. and Peterson, W. (1976). Various receptor sites in membrane fractions from corn coleoptiles: in vitro binding of auxins, riboflavin and a naturally occurring analog of morphactin. Abstr. 9th Int. Conf. Plant Growth Subst. (P.-E. Pilet, ed.). pp 140a-140c. Lausanne.

Hertel, R., Lomax, T.L. and Briggs, W.R. (1983). Auxin transport in membrane vesicles from Cucurbita pepo L. Planta 157, 193-201.

Hetherington, A.M. and Trewavas, A.J. (1984). Binding of nitrendipine, a calcium channel blocker, to pea shoot membranes. Plant Sci. Lett. 35, 109-113.

Higgins, T.J.V., Zwar, J.A. and Jacobsen, J.V. (1976). Gibberellic acid enhances the level of translatable mRNA for α-amylase in barley aleurone layers. Nature (London) 260, 166-169.

Hiraga, K., Yamane, H. and Takahashi, N. (1974). Biological activity of some synthetic gibberellin glucosyl esters. Phytochemistry 13, 2371-2376.

Ho, T.H.D., Shih, S.C. and Kleinhofs, A. (1980). Screening for barley mutants with altered hormone sensitivity in their aleurone layers. Plant Physiol. 68, 153-157.

Ho, T.H.D., Nolan, R.C. and Shute, D.E. (1981). Characterization of a gibberellin-insensitive dwarf wheat, D6899. Plant Physiol. 67, 1026-1031.

Hoad, G.V., Macmillan, J., Smith, V.A., Sponsel, V.M. and Taylor, D.A. (1982). Gibberellin 2β-hydroxylases and biological activity of 2β-alkyl gibberellins. In: 'Plant Growth Substances 1982'. (P.F. Wareing, ed.). pp 91-100. Academic Press, London - New York.

Hocking, T.J., Clapham, J. and Cattell, K.J. (1978). Abscisic acid binding to subcellular fractions from leaves of Vicia faba. Planta 138, 303-304.

Horgan, R., Hewett, E.W., Horgan, J.M., Purse, J. and Wareing, P.F. (1975). A new cytokinin from Populus robusta. Phytochemistry 14, 1005-1008.

Hornberg, C. and Weiler, E.W. (1984). High-affinity binding sites for abscisic acid on the plasmalemma of Vicia faba guard cells. Nature (London) 310, 321-324.

Hummel, J.P. and Dreyer, W.J. (1962). Measurement of protein-binding phenomena by gel filtration. Biochim. Biophys. Acta 63, 530-532.

Hunston, D.L. (1975). Two techniques for evaluating small molecule-macromolecule binding in complex systems. Anal. Biochem. 63, 99-109.

Ihl, M. (1976). Indole-acetic acid binding proteins in soybean cotyledon. Planta 131, 223-228.

Iwamura, H., Fujita, T., Koyama, S., Koshimiza, K. and Kumazawa, Z. (1980). Quantitative structure-activity relationship of cytokinin-active adenine and urea derivatives. Phytochemistry 19, 1309-1319.

Jablonovic, M. and Nooden, L.D. (1974). Changes in competable IAA binding in relation to bud development in pea seedlings. Plant Cell Physiol. 15, 687-692.

Jacobs, M. and Gilbert, S.F. (1983). Basal localisation of the presumptive auxin transport carrier in pea stem cells. Science 220, 1297-1300.

Jacobs, M. and Hertel, R. (1978). Auxin-binding to subcellular fractions from Cucurbita hypocotyls. Planta 142, 1-10.

Jacobsen, H.-J. (1982). Soluble auxin-binding proteins in pea epicotyls. Physiol. Plant. 56, 161-167.

Jacobsen, H.-J. (1984). Two different soluble cytoplasmic auxin-binding sites in etiolated pea epicotyls. Plant Cell Physiol. 25, 867-873.

Jacobsen, J.V. and Higgins, T.J.V. (1978). The influence of phytohormones on replication and transcription. In: 'Phytohormones and Related Compounds: A Comprehensive Treatise'. (D.S. Letham, P.B. Goodwin and T.J.V. Higgins, eds.). Vol. 1. pp 515-582. Elsevier Biomedical Press, Amsterdam - Oxford - New York.

Jacobsen, J.V., Chandler, P.M., Higgins, T.J.V. and Zwar, J.A. (1982). Control of protein synthesis in barley aleurone layers by gibberellin. In: 'Plant Growth Substances 1982'. (P.F. Wareing, ed.). pp 111-120. Academic Press, London - New York.

Janik, J.R. and Adler, J.H. (1984). Estrogen receptors in Gladiolus ovules. Plant Physiol. 75 S, 135.

Jelsema, C.L., Ruddat, M., Moore, D.J. and Williamson, F.A. (1977). Specific binding of gibberellin A_1 to aleurone grain fraction from wheat endosperm. Plant Cell Physiol. 18, 1009-1019.

Jerie, P.H., Shaari, A.R., Zeroni, M. and Hall, M.A. (1978). The partition coefficient of $^{14}C_2H_4$ in plant tissue as a screening test for metabolism or compartmentation of ethylene. New Phytol. 81, 499-504.

Jerie, P.H., Shaari, A.R. and Hall, M.A. (1979). The compartmentation of ethylene in developing cotyledons of Phaseolus vulgaris L. Planta 144, 503-507.

Johnson, L.P., MacLeod, J.K., Parker, C.W., Letham, D.S. and Hunt, N.H. (1981). Identification and quantitation of adenosine-3':5'-cyclic monophosphate in plants using gas chromatography-mass spectrometry and high-performance liquid chromatography. Planta 152, 195-201.

Johri, M.M. and Varner, J.E. (1968). Enhancement of RNA synthesis in isolated pea nuclei by gibberellic acid. Proc. Natl. Acad. Sci. USA 59, 260-276.

Jones, A.M., Melhado, L.L., Ho, T.H.D. and Leonard, N.J. (1984a). Azido auxins. Quantitative binding data in maize. Plant Physiol. 74, 295-301.

Jones, A.M., Melhado, L.L., Ho, T.H.D., Pearce, C.J., and Leonard, N.J. (1984b). Azido auxins: photaffinity labelling of auxin-binding proteins in maize coleoptile with tritiated 5-azidoindole-3-acetic acid. Plant Physiol. 75, 1111-1116.

Jones, G.P. and Paleg, L.E. (1984a). Complex formation between indole-3-acetic acid and phospholipid membrane components in aqueous media. 2. Interaction of auxins and related compounds with phosphatidylcholine membranes. Biochemistry 23, 1521-1524.

Jones, G.P. and Paleg, L.E. (1984b). Complex formation between indole-3-acetic acid and phospholipid membrane components in aqueous media. 3. Interaction of indole-3-acetic acid with amphiphiles containing the trimethylammonium group. Biochemistry 23, 1525-1532.

Jones, G.P., Marker, A. and Paleg, L.G. (1984). Complex formation between indole-3-acetic acid and phospholipid membrane components in aqueous media. 1. Parameters of the system. Biochemistry 23, 1514-1520.

Jönssen, A. (1961). Chemical structure and growth activity of auxins and antiauxins. In: 'Encyclopedia of Plant Physiology'. (W. Ruhland, ed.). Vol. XIV. pp 959-1006. Springer, Berlin - Göttingen - Heidelberg.

Kaethner, T.M. (1977). Conformational change theory for auxin structure-activity relationships. Nature (London) 267, 19-23.

Kasamo, K. and Yamaki, T. (1973). The stimulative effect of auxins in vitro on Mg^{++}-activated ATPase activity in crude enzyme extract from mung bean hypocotyls. Sci. Pap. Gen. Educ. Univ. Tokyo 23, 131-138.

Kasamo, K. and Yamaki, T. (1974). Effect of auxin on Mg^{++}-activated and inhibited ATPases from mung bean hypocotyls. Plant Cell Physiol. 15, 965-970.

Kasamo, K. and Yamaki, T. (1976). In vitro binding of IAA to plasma membrane-rich fractions containing Mg^{++}-activated ATPase from mung bean hypocotyls. Plant Cell Physiol. 17, 149-164.

Kasuga, M., Fujita-Yamaguchi, Y., Blithe, D.L. and Kahn, C.R. (1983). Tyrosine-specific protein kinase activity is associated with the purified insulin receptor. Proc. Natl. Acad. Sci. USA 80, 2137-2141.

Katekar, G.F. (1976). Inhibitors of the geotropic response in plants, a correlation of molecular structures. Phytochemistry 15, 1421-1424.

Katekar, G.F. (1979). Auxins: on the nature of the receptor site and molecular requirements for auxin activity. Phytochemistry 18, 223-233.

Katekar, G.F. (1985). Interaction of phytotropins with the NPA receptor. Biol. Plantarum (in press).

Katekar, G.F. and Geissler, A.E. (1975). Auxin transport inhibitors: fluorescein and related compounds. Plant Physiol. 56, 645-646.

Katekar, G.F. and Geissler, A.E. (1977). Auxin transport inhibitors. III. Chemical requirements of a class of auxin transport inhibitors. Plant Physiol. 80, 826-829.

Katekar, G.F. and Geissler, A.E. (1980). Auxin transport inhibitors. IV. Evidence of a common mode of action for a proposed class of auxin transport inhibitors, the phytotropins. Plant Physiol. 66, 1190-1195.

Katekar, G.F. and Geissler, A.E. (1981). Phytotropins: conformational requirements for the abolition of the root geotropic response. Phytochemistry 20, 2465-2469.

Katekar, G.F. and Geissler, A.E. (1983). Structure-activity differences between indoleacetic acid auxins on pea and wheat. Phytochemistry 22, 27-31.

Katekar, G.F., Navé, J.F., and Geissler, A.E. (1981). Phytotropins III. Naphthylphthalamic acid binding sites on maize coleoptile membranes as possible receptor sites for phytotropin action. Plant Physiol. 68, 1460-1464.

Kato, J., Katsumi, M. Tamura, S. and Sakurai, A. (1968). Plant growth-regulating activities of helminthosporol and its derivatives. In: 'Biochemistry and Physiology of Plant Growth Substances'. (F. Wightman, G. Setterfield, eds.). pp 347-359. Runge Press, Ottawa.

Kearns, A.W. (1982). The search for the auxin receptor. D.Phil. thesis, University of York.

Keates, R.A.B. (1973). Evidence that cyclic AMP does not mediate the action of gibberellic acid. Nature (London) 244, 355-357.

Kefford, N.P., Zwar, J.A. and Bruce, M.I. (1968). Antagonism of purine and urea cytokinin activities by derivatives of benzylurea. In: 'Biochemistry and Physiology of Plant Growth Substances'. (F. Wightman and G. Setterfield, eds.). pp 61-69. Runge Press, Ottawa.

Keim, P. and Fox, J.E. (1980). Interaction of a radiolabeled cytokinin photoaffinity probe with a receptor protein. Biochem. Biophys. Res. Commun. 96, 1325-1334.

Keim, P., Erion, J. and Fox, J.E. (1981). The current status of cytokinin-binding moieties. In: 'Metabolism and Molecular Activities of Cytokinins'. (J. Guern and C. Peaud-Lenoel, eds.). pp 179-190. Springer-Verlag, Berlin.

Keith, B. and Srivastava, L.M. (1980). In vivo binding of gibberellin A_1 in dwarf pea epicotyls. Plant Physiol. 66, 962-967.

Keith, B., Boal, R. and Srivastava, L.M. (1980). On the uptake, metabolism and retention of ^3H gibberellin A_1 by barley aleurone layers at low temperatures. Plant Physiol. 66, 956-961.

Keith, B., Foster, N.A. and Srivastava, L.M. (1981). In vitro gibberellin A_4 binding to extracts of cucumber hypocotyls. Plant Physiol. 68, 344-348.

Keith, B., Brown, S. and Srivastava, L.M. (1982). In vitro binding of gibberellin A_4 to extracts of cucumber measured by using DEAE-cellulose filters. Proc. Natl. Acad. Sci. USA 79, 1515-1519.

Keith, B., Thompson, R.H. and Rappaport, L. (1984). ^3H gibberellin A_1 binding to extracts of corn leaf sheaths. Plant Physiol. 75 S, 92.

Kende, H. and Gardner, G. (1976). Hormone binding in plants. Ann. Rev. Plant. Physiol. 27, 267-290.

Kennedy, C.D. (1971). A new model membrane system for the investigation of penetrative properties of plant growth substances. Pestic. Sci. 2, 69-74.

Kennedy, C.D. and Harvey, J.M. (1972). Plant growth substance action on lecithin and lecithin/cholesterol vesicles. Pestic. Sci. 3, 715-727.

Kerk, G.J.M. van der, Raalte, M.H. van, Sijpesteijn, A.K. and Veen, R. van der (1955). A new type of plant growth regulating substance. Nature (London) 176, 308-310.

Kharchenko, V.I., Romanko, E.G., Selivankina, S.Y. and Kulaeva, O.N. (1984). Isolation of cytokinin-binding proteins from barley leaves by means of affinity chromatography. Soviet Plant Physiol. 30, 932-936.

King, W.J. and Greene, G.L. (1984). Monoclonal antibodies localize oestrogen receptor in the nuclei of target cells. Nature (London) 307, 745-747.

Klun, J.A., Tipton, C.L., Robinson, J.F., Ostrem, D.L., and Beroza, M. (1970). Isolation and identification of 6,7-dimethoxy-2-benzoxazolinone from dried tissues of Zea mays (L.) and evidence of its cyclic hydroxamic acid precursor. J. Agric. Food Chem. 18, 663-665.

Knöfel, H.D., Müller, P., Kramell, R. and Sembdner, G. (1975). Preparation of gibberellin affinity adsorbents. FEBS Letters 60, 39-41.

Kobayashi, K., Zbell, B. and Reinert, J. (1981). A high affinity binding site for cytokinin to a particulate fraction in carrot suspension cells. Protoplasma 106, 145-155.

Koenig, H., Goldstone, A. and Lu, C-Y. (1983). Polamines regulate calcium fluxes in a rapid plasma membrane response. Nature (London) 305, 530-534.

Koepfli, J.B., Thimann, K.V. and Went, F.W. (1938). Phytohormones: structure and physiological activity. J. Biol. Chem. 122, 763-780.

Konjevic, R., Grubisic, D., Markovic, R. and Petrovic, J. (1976). Gibberellic acid binding proteins from pea stems. Planta 131, 125-128.

Koornneef, M., Reuling, G. and Karssen, C.M. (1984). The isolation and characterization of abscisic acid-insensitive mutants of Arabidopsis thaliana. Physiol. Plant. 61, 377-383.

Kubowicz, B.D., Vanderhoef, L.N. and Hanson, J.B. (1982). ATP-dependent calcium transport in plasmalemma preparations from soybean hypocotyls. Plant Physiol. 69, 187-191.

Kyriakidis, D.A. (1983). Effect of plant growth hormones and polyamines on ornithine decarboxylase activity during the germination of barley seeds. Physiol. Plant. 57, 499-504.

Lado, P., Cerana, R., Bonetti, A., Marrè, M.T. and Marrè, E. (1981). Effects of calmodulin inhibitors in plants I. Synergism with fusicoccin in the stimulation of growth and H^+ secretion. Plant Sci. Lett. 23, 253-262.

Lehmann, P.A. (1978). Stereoselectivity and affinity in molecular pharmacology III. Structural aspects in the mode of action of natural and synthetic auxins. Chem. Biol. Interactions 20, 239-249.

LeJohn, H.B. (1975). A rapid and sensitive binding system for N^6-substituted adenines, and some urea and thiourea derivatives, that show cytokinin activity in cell division tests. Can. J. Biochem. 53, 768-775.

Lembi, C.A., Morré, D.J., Thomson, K.-St., and Hertel, R. (1971). N-1-naphthylphthalamic-acid-binding activity of a plasma membrane-rich fraction from maize coleoptiles. Planta 99, 37-45.

Leonard, N.J., Greenfield, J.C., Schmitz, R.Y. and Skoog, F. (1975). Photoaffinity-labelled auxins. Plant Physiol. 55, 1057-1061.

Letham, D.S. (1978). Cytokinins. In: 'Phytohormones and Related Compounds: A Comprehensive Treatise'. (D.S. Letham, P.B. Goodwin and T.J.V. Higgins, eds.). Vol. 1, pp 205-263. Elsevier Biomedical Press, Amsterdam - Oxford - New York.

Likholat, T.V., Pospelov, V.A., Morozova, T.M. and Salganik, R.I. (1974). Capacity of wheat coleoptile cells for specific binding of auxin and effect of the hormone on template activity of chromatin in seedlings of different ages. Sov. Plant Physiol. 21, 779-784.

Lin, P.P.C. (1974). Cyclic nucleotides in higher plants? Adv. Cyclic Nucleotide Res. 4, 439-461.

Lin, P.P.C. (1984). Polamine metabolism and its relation to response of the aleurone layers of barley seed to gibberellic acid. Plant Physiol. 74, 975-983.

Linsley, P.S., Das, M. and Fox, C.F. (1981). Affinity labelling of hormone receptors and other ligand binding proteins. In: 'Receptors and Recognition'. (S. Jacobs and P. Cuatrecasas, eds.). Series B Vol. 11. pp 89-113. Chapman and Hall, London.

Löbler, M., and Klämbt, D. (1984). Purification and characterization of an auxin-binding protein from maize coleoptiles with immunological methods. Abstracts, 16th FEBS Meeting Moscow, p 427.

Lomax, T.L. and Mehlhorn, R.J. (1985). Determination of osmotic volumes and pH gradients of plant membrane and lipid vesicles using ESR spectroscopy. Biochim. Biophys. Acta (in press).

Lomax, T.L., Mehlhorn, R.J. and Briggs, W.R. (1985). Active auxin uptake by zucchini membrane vesicles: quantitation using ESR volume and Δ pH measurements. Proc. Natl. Acad. Sci. USA (in press).

Lomax-Reichert, T., Ashton, N.W. and Ray, P.M. (1982). Naphthaleneacetic acid and fusicoccin binding to membrane fractions of the moss Physcomitrella patens. In: 'Plasmalemma and Tonoplast: Their Functions in the Plant Cell'. (D. Marme, E. Marre and R. Hertel, eds.). pp 303-310. Elsevier Biomedical Press, Amsterdam - New York - Oxford.

Maan, A.C., Vreugdenhil, D., Bogers, R.J. and Libbenga, K.R. (1983). The complex kinetics of auxin-binding to a particulate fraction from tobacco pith callus. Planta 158, 10-15.

Maan, A.C., Kühnel, B., Benkers, J.J.B. and Libbenga, K.R. (1985a). Naphthylphthalamic acid binding sites in cultured cells from Nicotiana tabacum. Planta 164, 69-74..

Maan, A.C., Van der Linde, P.C.G., Harkes, P.A.A. and Libbenga, K.R. (1985b). Correlation between the presence of membrane-bound auxin binding and root regeneration in cultured tobacco cells. Planta (in press).

Maher, E.P. and Martindale, S.J.B. (1980). Mutants of Arabidopsis thaliana with altered responses to auxins and gravity. Biochem. Genet. 18, 1041-1053.

Malmberg, R.L. and McIndoo, J. (1983). Abnormal floral development of a tobacco mutant with elevated polyamine levels. Nature (London) 305, 623-625.

Marrè, E. (1979). Fusicoccin: a tool in plant physiology. Ann. Rev. Plant Physiol. 30, 273-288.

Matthysse, A.G. (1970). Organ specificity of hormone receptor-chromatin interactions. Biochim. Biophys. Acta 199, 519-521.

Matthysse, A.G. and Abrams, M. (1970). A factor mediating interaction of kinins with the genetic material. Biochim. Biophys. Acta 199, 511-518.

Matthysse, A.G. and Phillips, C. (1969). A protein intermediary in the interaction of a hormone with the genome. Proc. Natl. Acad. Sci. USA 63, 897-903.

Melhado, L.L., Jones, A.M., Leonard, N.J. and Vanderhoef, L.N. (1981). Azido auxins: synthesis and biological activity of fluorescent photoaffinity labelling agents. Plant Physiol. 68, 469-475.

Melhado, L.L., Jones, A.M., Ho, T.-H.D. and Leonard, N.J. (1984). Azido auxins. Photolysis in solution and covalent binding to soybean. Plant Physiol. 74, 289-294.

Melton, D.A. (1985). Injected anti-sense RNAs specifically block messenger RNA translation in vivo. Proc. Natl. Acad. Sci. USA 82, 144-148.

Mertens, R. and Weiler, E.W. (1983). Kinetic studies on the redistribution of endogenous growth regulators in gravireacting plant organs. Planta 158, 339-348.

Mertens, R. Stüning, M. and Weiler, E.W. (1982). Metabolism of tritiated enantiomers of abscisic acid prepared by immunoaffinity chromatography. Naturwiss. 69, 595-597.

Milborrow, B.V. (1974). The chemistry and physiology of abscisic acid. Ann. Rev. Plant Physiol. 25, 259-307.

Milborrow, B.V. (1978). Abscisic acid. In: 'Phytohormones and Related Compounds: A Comprehensive Treatise'. (D.S. Letham, P.G. Goodwin and T.J.V. Higgins, eds.). Vol. 1. pp 295-347. Elsevier Biomedical Press, Amsterdam - Oxford - New York.

Mitchell, J.W. Mandava, N., Worley, J.F., Plummer, J.R. and Smith, M.V. (1970). Brassins - a new family of plant hormones from rape pollen. Nature (London) 225, 1065-1066.

Moloney, M.M. and Pilet, P.E. (1981). Auxin binding in roots: a comparison between maize roots and coleoptiles. Planta 153, 447-452.

Moloney, M.M. and Pilet, P.E. (1982). Auxin binding in root tissues. Abstracts, Eleventh International Conference on Plant Growth Substances, Aberystwyth, p 24.

Moloney, M.M., Henri, H. and Pilet, P.E. (1983). Regulation of in vitro H$^+$-transport in sealed pea root vesicles. Plant Physiol. 72 S, 140.

Mondal, H., Mandal, R.K. and Biswas, B.B. (1972). RNA stimulated by indole acetic acid. Nature (London) New Biol. 240, 111-112.

Monod, J., Changeux, J.-P. and Jacob, F. (1963). Alosteric proteins and cellular control systems. J. Mol. Biol. 6, 306-329.

Moore, F.H. (1979). A cytokinin-binding protein from wheat germ. Plant Physiol. 64, 594-599.

Mornet, R., Theiler, J.B., Leonard, N.J., Schmitz, R.Y., Moore, F.H. and Skoog, F. (1979). Active cytokinins. Photoaffinity labeling agents to detect binding. Plant Physiol. 64, 600-610.

Morré, D.J. and Bracker, C.E. (1976). Ultrastructural alteration of plant plasma membranes induced by auxin and calcium ions. Plant Physiol. 58, 544-547.

Morré, D.J., Morre, J.T. and Varnold, R.L. (1984). Phosphorylation of membrane-located proteins of soybean in vitro and response to auxin. Plant Physiol. 75, 265-268.

Morré, D.J., Gripshover, B., Monroe, A. and Morré, J.T. (1984). Phosphatidylinositol turnover in isolated soybean membranes stimulated by the synthetic growth hormone 2,4-dichlorophenoxyacetic acid. J. Biol. Chem. 259, 15364-15368.

Muir, R.M., Hansch, C. and Gallup, A.H. (1949). Growth regulation by organic compounds. Plant Physiol. 24, 359-366.

Munson, P.J. and Rodbard, D. (1980). LIGAND: A versatile computerized approach for characterization of ligand-binding systems. Anal. Biochem. 107, 220-239.

Murphy, G.J.P. (1979). Plant hormone receptors: comparison of naphthaleneacetic acid binding by maize extracts and by a non-plant protein. Plant Sci. Lett. 16, 115-121.

Murphy, G.J.P. (1980a). A reassessment of the binding of naphthaleneacetic acid by membrane preparations from maize. Planta 149, 417-426.

Murphy, G.J.P. (1980b). Naphthaleneacetic acid binding by membrane-free preparations of cytosol from the maize coleoptile. Plant Sci. Lett. 19, 157-168.

Murray, M.G. and Key, J.L. (1978). 2,4-dichlorophenoxyacetic acid-enhanced phosphorylation of soybean nuclear proteins. Plant Physiol. 61, 190-198.

Muthukrishnan, S., Chandra, G.R. and Maxwell, E.S. (1983). Hormonal control of α-amylase gene expression in barley. J. Biol. Chem. 258, 2370-2375.

Narayanan, K.R., Mudge, K.W. and Poovaiah, B.W. (1981a). In vitro auxin binding to cellular membranes of cucumber fruits. Plant Physiol. 67, 836-840.

Narayanan, K.R., Mudge, K.W. and Poovaiah, B.W. (1981b). Demonstration of auxin binding to strawberry fruit membranes. Plant Physiol. 68, 1289-1293.

Navé, J.-F. and Benveniste, P. (1984). Inactivation by phenylglyoxal of the specific binding of 1-naphthyl acetic acid with membrane-bound auxin binding sites from maize coleoptiles. Plant Physiol. 74, 1035-1040.

Newton, R.P., Gibbs, N., Moyse, C.D., Wiebers, J.L. and Brown, E.G. (1980). Mass spectrometric identification of adenosine 3':5'-cyclic monophosphate isolated from a higher plant tissue. Phytochemistry 19, 1909-1911.

Nicholls, S.E. and Laties, G.G. (1984). Ethylene-regulated gene transcription in carrot roots. Plant Mol. Biol. 3, 393-401.

Normand, G., Hartman, M.A., Schuber, F. and Benveniste, P. (1975). Charactérisation de membranes de coléoptiles de mais fixant l'auxine et l'acide N-naphtyl phtalmique. Physiol. Vég. 13, 743-761.

Normand, G., Schuber, F., Benveniste, P. and Beauvais, D. (1977). Effect of red light on the binding of NAA on maize coleoptile membranes. In: 'Regulation of Cell Membrane Activities in Plants'. (E. Marrè and O. Ciferri, eds.). pp 225-230. Elsevier Biomedical Press, Amsterdam.

Obata, T., Taniguchi, H. and Maruyama, Y. (1983). The effect of calmodulin antagonists on gibberellic acid-induced enzyme secretion in barley aleurone layers. Ann. Bot. 52, 877-883.

O'Brien, T.J., Jarvis, B.C., Cherry, J.H. and Hanson, J.B. (1968). Enhancement by 2,4-D of chromatin RNA polymerase in soybean hypocotyl tissue. Biochim. Biophys. Acta 169, 35-43.

Okamoto, T., Isogai, Y. and Koizumi, T. (1967). Isolation of indole-3-acetic acid, phenylacetic acid and several plant growth inhibitors from etiolated seedlings of Phaseolus. Chem. Pharm. Bull. 15, 159-163.

Olah, Z., Berczi, A. and Erdei, L. (1983). Benzylaminopurine-induced coupling between calmodulin and Ca-ATPase in wheat root microsomal membranes. FEBS Lett. 154, 395-399.

O'Malley, B. and Means, A.R. (1974). Female steroid hormones and target cell nuclei. Science 183, 610-620.

Oostrom, H., Van Loopik-Detmers, M.A., and Libbenga, K.R. (1975). A high affinity receptor for indoleacetic acid in cultured tobacco pith explants. FEBS Lett. 59, 194-197.

Oostrom, H., Kulescha, Z., Van Vliet, T.B. and Libbenga, K.R. (1980). Characterization of a cytoplasmic auxin receptor from tobacco-pith callus. Planta 149, 44-47.

Oritz de Montellano, P.R., Beilan, H.S., Kunze, K.L. and Mico, B.A. (1981). Destruction of cytochrome P-450 by ethylene - Structure of the resulting prosthetic heme adduct. J. Biol. Chem. 256, 4395-4399.

Paleg, L.G., Wood, A. and Spotswood, T.M. (1974). Interaction of GA_3 and IAA with a natural plant constituent. In: 'Plant Growth Substances 1973'. pp 732-736. Hirokawa, Tokyo.

Pauls, K.P., Chambers, J.A., Dumbroff, E.B. and Thompson, J.E. (1982). Perturbation of phospholipid membranes by gibberellins. New Phytol. 91, 1-17.

Paulus, H. (1969). A rapid and sensitive method for measuring the binding of radioactive ligands to proteins. Anal. Biochem. 32, 91-100.

Pearson, J.A. and Wareing, P.F. (1969). Effect of abscisic acid on activity of chromatin. Nature (London) 221, 672-673.

Penny, P. and Penny, D. (1978). Rapid responses to phytohormones. In: 'Phytohormones and Related Compounds. A Comprehensive Treatise'. (D.S. Letham, P.B. Goodwin and T.J.V. Higgins, eds.). Vol. II, pp 537-597. Elsevier Biomedical Press, Amsterdam - Oxford - New York.

Penny, P., Penny, D., Marshall, D. and Heyes, J.K. (1972). Early responses of excised stem sections to auxins. J. Exp. Bot. 23, 23-36.

Pesci, P. Cocucci, S.M. and Randazzo, G. (1979a). Characterization of fusicoccin binding to receptor sites on cell membranes of maize coleoptile tissues. Plant, Cell Environment 2, 205-209.

Pesci, P., Tognoli, L. Beffagna, N. and Marrè, E. (1979b). Solubilization and partial purification of a fusicoccin-receptor complex from maize microsomes. Plant Sci. Lett. 15, 313-322.

Petruzzelli, L., Herrera, R. and Rosen, O.M. (1984). Insulin receptor is an insulin-dependent tyrosine protein kinase. Proc. Natl. Acad. Sci. USA 81, 3327-3331.

Phinney, B.O. and Spray, C. (1982). Chemical genetics and the gibberellin pathway in Zea mays. In: 'Plant Growth Substances 1982'. (P.F. Wareing, ed.). pp 101-110. Academic Press, London - New York.

Polya, G.M. and Bowman, J.A. (1979). Ligand specificity of a high affinity cytokinin-binding protein. Plant Physiol. 64, 387-392.

Polya, G.M. and Davies, J.R. (1983). Resolution and properties of a protein kinase catalyzing the phosphorylation of a wheat germ cytokinin-binding protein. Plant Physiol. 71, 482-488.

Polya, G.M. and Davis, A.W. (1978). Properties of a high-affinity cytokinin-binding protein from wheat germ. Planta 139, 139-147.

Porter, W.L. and Thimann, K.V. (1959). Molecular and functional complementarity of auxins and phosphatides. Abstr. 9th Int. Bot. Congr. Vol. II. pp 305-306. University of Toronto Press.

Porter, W.L. and Thimann, K.V. (1965). Molecular requirements for auxin action. I. Halogenated indoles and indoleacetic acid. Phytochemistry 4, 229-243.

Qi, D.-F., Schatzmann, R.C., Mazzei, G.Z., Turner, R.S., Raynor, R.L., Liao, S. and Kuo, J.F. (1983). Polyamines inhibit phospholipid-sensitive and calmodulin-sensitive Ca^{2+}-dependent protein kinases. Biochem. J. 213, 281-288.

Quail, P.H. and Browning, A. (1977). Failure of lactoperoxidase to iodinate specifically the plasma membrane of Cucurbita tissue segments. Plant Physiol. 59, 759-766.

Radice, M., Scacchi, A., Pesci, P., Beffagna, N. and Marrè, M.T. (1981). Comparative analysis of the effects of fusicoccin and of its derivative dideacetylfusicoccin on maize leaves and roots. Physiol. Plant. 51, 215-221.

Rakhaminova, A.B., Kharkin, E.E. and Yaguzhinskii, L.S. (1978). Construction of a model of the auxin receptor. Dokl. Biochem. 43, 639-653.

Ranjeva, R., Refeno, G., Boudet, A.M. and Marmé, D. (1983). Activation of plant quinate:NAD^+3-oxidoreductase by Ca^{2+} and calmodulin. Proc. Natl. Acad. Sci. USA 80, 5222-5224.

Ray, P.M. (1977). Auxin binding sites of maize coleoptiles are localized on membranes of the endoplasmic reticulum. Plant Physiol. 59, 594-599.

Ray, P.M., Dohrmann, V., and Hertel, R. (1977a). Characterization of naphthaleneacetic acid binding to receptor sites on cellular membranes of maize coleoptiles tissue. Plant Physiol. 59, 357-364.

Ray, P.M., Dohrmann, U., and Hertel, R. (1977b). Specificity of auxin-binding sites on maize coleoptile membranes as possible receptor sites for auxin action. Plant Physiol. 60, 585-591.

Rayle, D.L. (1973). Auxin-induced H^+-ion secretion in Avena coleoptiles and its implications. Planta 114, 63-73.

Reddy, A.S.N., Sopory, S.K. and Datta, A. (1983). Purification and characterization of a cytokinin binding protein from barley embryos. Biochem. International 6, 181-190.

Reeve, D.R. and Crozier, A. (1974). An assessment of gibberellin structure-activity relationships. J. Exp. Bot. 25, 431-445.

Rizzo, P.J., Pederson, K. and Cherry, J.H. (1977). Stimulation of transcription by a soluble factor isolated from soybean hypocotyl by 2,4-D affinity chromatography. Plant Sci. Lett. 8, 205-211.

Roberts, D.D. and Goldstein, I.J. (1983). Adenine binding sites of the lectin from lima beans. J. Biol. Chem. 258, 13820-13824.

Robichand, C.S., Wong, J. and Sussex, I.M. (1980). Control of in vitro growth of viviporous embryo mutants of maize by abscisic acid. Dev. Genetics 1, 325-330.

Robison, G.A., Butcher, R.W. and Sutherland, E.W. (1968). Cyclic AMP. Ann. Rev. Biochem. 37, 149-174.

Romanko, E.G., Selivankina, S.Y., Kuroedov, V.A., Kharchenko, V.I. and Kulaeva, O.N. (1982). Functional activity of cytokinin-binding proteins from barley leaves and pumpkin cotyledons. Dokl. Bot. Sci. 267, 137-139.

Roy, P. and Biswas, B.B. (1977). A receptor protein for indoleacetic acid from plant chromatin and its role in transcription. Biochem. Biophys. Res. Commun. 74, 1597-1606.

Rubery, P.H. (1981). Auxin receptors. Ann. Rev. Plant Physiol. 32, 569-596.

Rubery, P.H. and Sheldrake, A.R. (1974). Carrier-mediated auxin transport. Planta 118, 101-121.

Rubinstein, B. (1982). Regulation of H^+ excretion. Role of protein released by osmotic shock. Plant Physiol. 69, 945-949.

Sakai, S. (1984). Characterization of 2,4-D binding to the auxin-binding protein purified from etiolated mung bean seedlings. Agric. Biol. Chem. 48, 257-259.

Sakai, S. and Hanagata, T. (1983). Purification of an auxin-binding protein from etiolated mung bean seedlings by affinity chromatography. Plant Cell Physiol. 24, 685-693.

Scatchard, G. (1949). The attractions of proteins for small molecules and ions. Ann. N.Y. Acad. Sci. 51, 660-672.

Scherer, G.F.E. (1981). Auxin-stimulated ATPase in membrane fractions from pumpkin hypocotyls. Planta 151, 434-438.

Scherer, G.F.E. (1984a). Stimulation of ATPase activity by auxin is dependent on ATP concentration. Planta 161, 394-397.

Scherer, G.F.E. (1984b). H⁺-ATPase and auxin-stimulated ATPase in membrane fractions from zucchini and pumpkin hypocotyls. Z. Pflanz. 114, 233-237.

Scherer, G.F.E. and Morré, D.J. (1978). In vitro stimulation by 2,4-dichlorophenoxyacetic acid of an ATPase and inhibition of phosphatidate phosphatase of plant membranes. Biochem. Biophys. Res. Commun. 84, 238-247.

Schneider, J.A., Yoshihara, K., Nakanishi, K. and Kato, N. (1983). Typhasterol (2-deoxycastasterone): a new plant growth regulator from cat-tail pollen. Tetrahedron Lett. 24, 3859-3860.

Selivankina, S.Y., Romanko, E.G., Ovcharov, A.K. and Kharchenko, V.I. (1982a). Participation of cytokinin-binding proteins from barley leaves in cytokinin activation of chromatin-bound RNA polymerase. Sov. Plant Physiol. 29, 208-214.

Selivankina, S.Y., Romanko, E.G., Kuroedov, V.A., Karavaiko, N.N. and Kulaeva, O.N. (1982b). Activation of barley leaf RNA polymerase in vitro by cytokinin-receptor complex. Dokl. Bot. Sci. 267, 132-134.

Sembdner, G., Gross, D., Liebisch, H.-W. and Schneider, G. (1980). Biosynthesis and metabolism of plant hormones. In: 'Encyclopedia of Plant Physiology, N.S. Vol. 9: Hormonal Regulation of Development'. (J. MacMillan, ed.). pp 281-444. Springer-Verlag, Berlin - Heidelberg - New York.

Serebryakov, E.P., Agnistikova, V.N. and Suslova, L.M. (1984a). Growth-promoting activity of some selectively modified gibberellins. Phytochemistry 23, 1847-1854.

Serebryakov, E.P., Epstein, N.A. Yasinskaya, N.P. and Kaplun, A.B. (1984b). A mathematical additive model of the structure-activity relationships of gibberellins. Phytochemistry 23, 1855-1863.

Shantz, E.M. and Steward, F.C. (1955). The identification of compound A from coconut milk as 1,3-diphenylurea. J. Am. Chem. Soc. 77, 6351-6353.

Siegel, S.M. and Galston, A.W (1953). Experimental coupling of indoleacetic acid to pea root protein in vivo and in vitro. Proc. Natl. Acad. Sci. USA 39, 1111-1118.

Singh, S.P. and Paleg, L.G. (1984). Low temperature induction of hormonal sensitivity in genotypically gibberellic acid-insensitive aleurone tissue. Plant Physiol. 74, 437-438.

Sisler, E.C. (1977). Ethylene activity of some π-acceptor compounds. Tob. Sci. 21, 43-45.

Sisler, E.C. (1979). Measurement of ethylene binding in plant tissue. Plant Physiol. 64, 538-542.

Sisler, E.C. (1980). Partial purification of an ethylene-binding component from plant tissue. Plant Physiol. 66, 404-406.

Sisler, E.C. (1982a). Ethylene-binding properties of a Triton X-100 extract of mung bean sprouts. J. Plant Growth Regul. 1, 211-218.

Sisler, E.C. (1982b). Ethylene binding in normal, rin, and nor mutant tomatoes. J. Plant Growth Regul. 1, 219-226.

Sisler, E.C. (1984). Distribution and properties of ethylene-binding component from plant tissue. In: 'Ethylene: Biochemical, Physiological and Applied Aspects'. (Y. Fuchs and E. Chalutz, eds.). pp 45-54. Martinus Nijhoff/Dr. W. Junk, The Hague.

Sisler, E.C. and Yang, S.F. (1984a). Ethylene, the gaseous plant hormone. BioScience 34, 234-238.

Sisler, E.C. and Yang, S.F. (1984b). Anti-ethylene effects of cis-2-butene and cyclic olefins. Phytochemistry 12, 2765-2768.

Sisler, E.C., Reid, M.S. and Yang, S.F. (1985). Effect of antagonists of ethylene action on binding of ethylene in cut carnations. Plant Growth Regul. (submitted).

Skoog, F., Schmitz, R.Y., Bock, R.M. and Hecht, S.M. (1973). Cytokinin antagonists: synthesis and physiological effects of 7-substituted-3-methylpyrazolo (4,3-d) pyrimidines. Phytochemistry 12, 25-37.

Slone, J.H. and Bilderback, D.F. (1983). Membrane-bound auxin binding sites in Alaska pea stems. Plant Physiol. 72 S, 116.

Slone, J.H. and Bilderback, D.F. (1984). In vitro uptake of indoleacetic acid into membrane vesicles from etiolated pea stems. Plant Physiol. 75 S, 111.

Smith, A.R. and Hall, M.A. (1984). Mechanisms of ethylene action. Plant Growth Regul. 2, 151-165.

Smith, A.R. and Hall, M.A. (1985). Ethylene binding. In: 'Ethylene and Plant Development'. (J.A. Roberts and G.A. Tucker, eds.). pp 101-116. Butterworths, London.

Smith, M.S., Wain, R.L. and Wightman, F. (1952). Studies of plant growth-regulating substances V. Steric factors in relation to mode of action of certain aryloxyalkylcarboxylic acids. Ann. Appl. Biol. 39, 295-307.

Smith, P.G., Venis, M.A. and Hall, M.A. (1985). Oxidation of ethylene by cotyledon extracts from Vicia faba L. Planta 163, 97-104.

Stillwell, W. and Hester, P. (1983). Kinetin increases water permeability
    of phosphatidylcholine lipid bilayers. Plant Physiol. 71, 524-530.

Stoddart, J.L. (1979a). Interaction of {^{3}H} gibberellin A$_1$ with a sub-
    cellular fraction from lettuce (Lactuca sativa L.) hypocotyls. I.
    Kinetics of labelling. Planta 146, 353-361.

Stoddart, J.L. (1979b). Interaction of {^{3}H} gibberellin A$_1$ with a sub-
    cellular fraction from lettuce (Lactuca sativa L.) hypocotyls. II.
    Stability and properties of the association. Planta 146, 363-368.

Stoddart, J.L. (1982). Gibberellin perception and its primary consequences.
    In: 'Plant Growth Substances 1982'. (P.F. Wareing, ed.). pp 131-140.
    Academic Press, London - New York.

Stoddart, J.L. and Venis, M.A. (1980). Molecular and subcellular aspects of
    hormone action. In: 'Encyclopedia of Plant Physiology, N.S., vol. 9:
    Hormonal Regulation of Development'. (J. MacMillan, ed.). pp 445-510.
    Springer-Verlag, Berlin - Heidelberg - New York.

Stoddart, J.L. and Williams, P.D. (1979). Interaction of {^{3}H} gibberellin
    A$_1$ with a sub-cellular fraction from lettuce (Lactuca sativa L.)
    hypocotyls. Requirement for protein synthesis. Planta 147, 264-268.

Stoddart, J.L. (1980). Interaction of {^{3}H} gibberellin A$_1$ with a
    subcellular fraction from lettuce (Lactuca sativa L.) hypocotyls. The
    relationship between growth and incorporation. Planta 148, 485-490.

Stoddart, J.L., Briedenbach, W., Nadau, R. and Rappaport, L. (1974).
    Selective binding of {^{3}H} gibberellin A$_1$ by protein fractions from dwarf
    pea epicotyls. Proc. Natl. Acad. Sci. USA 71, 3255-3259.

Stout, R.G. and Cleland, R.E. (1980). Partial characterization of
    fusicoccin binding to receptor sites on oat root membranes. Plant
    Physiol. 66, 353-359.

Strickland, S. and Loeb, J.N. (1981). Obligatory separation of hormone
    binding and biological response curves in systems dependent upon
    secondary mediators of hormone action. Proc. Natl. Acad. Sci. USA 78,
    1366-1370.

Strosberg, A.D. (1984). Receptors and recognition: from ligand binding to
    gene structure. Trends Biochem. Sci. 9, 166-169.

Südi, J. (1964). Induction of the formation of complexes between aspartic
    acid and indolyl-3-acetic acid or 1-naphthaleneacetic acid by other
    carboxylic acids. Nature (London) 201, 1009-1010.

Südi, J. (1966). Increases in the capacity of pea tissue to form acyl-
    aspartic acids specifically induced by auxins. New Phytol. 65, 9-21.

Sussman, M.R. and Gardner, G. (1980). Solubilisation of the receptor for N-
    naphthylphthalamic acid. Plant Physiol. 66, 1074-1078.

Sussman, M.R. and Goldsmith, M.H.M. (1981). The action of specific
inhibitors of auxin transport on uptake of auxin and binding of N-1-
naphthylphthalamic acid. Planta 152, 13-18.

Sussman, M.R. and Kende, H. (1977). The synthesis and biological properties
of 8-azido-N^6-benzyl-adenine, a potential photoaffinity reagent for
cytokinins. Planta 137, 91-96.

Sussman, M.R. and Kende, H. (1978). In vitro cytokinin binding to a
particulate fraction of tobacco cells. Planta 140, 251-259.

Sutherland, E.W. (1972). Studies on the mechanism of hormone action.
Science 177. 401-408.

Takatsuto, S., Yazawa, N., Ikekawa, N., Takematsu, T., Takeuchi, Y. and
Koguchi, M. (1983). Structure-activity relationship of brassinosteroids.
Phytochemistry 22, 2437-2441.

Takegami, T. and Yoshida, K. (1975). Isolation and purification of a
cytokinin binding protein from tobacco leaves by affinity column
chromatography. Biochem. Biophys. Res. Commun. 67, 782-789.

Takegami, T. and Yoshida, K. (1977). Specific interaction of cytokinin
binding protein with 40S ribosomal subunits in the presence of cytokinin
in vitro. Plant Cell Physiol. 18, 337-345.

Tappeser, B., Wellnitz, D., and Klämbt, D. (1981). Auxin affinity proteins
prepared by affinity chromatography. Z. Pflanzenphysiol. 101, 295-302.

Teissere, M., Penon, P. and Ricard, J. (1973). Hormonal control of
chromatin availability and of the activity of purified RNA polymerases in
higher plants. FEBS Lett. 30, 65-70.

Teissere, M. Penon, P., Van Huystee, R.B., Azou, Y. and Ricard, J. (1975).
Hormonal control of transcription in higher plants. Biochim. Biophys.
Acta. 402, 391-402.

Theiler, J.B., Leonard, N.J., Schmitz, R.Y. and Skoog, F. (1976).
Photoaffinity-labeled cytokinins. Plant Physiol. 58, 803-805.

Theologis, A. and Ray, P.M. (1982). Change in messenger RNAs under the
influence of auxins. In: 'Plant Growth Substances 1982'. (P.F. Wareing,
ed.). pp 43-57. Academic Press, London - New York.

Thimann, K.V. and Sweeney, B.M. (1937). The effect of auxins upon
protoplasmic streaming. J. gen. Physiol. 21, 123-135.

Thomas, C.J.R., Smith, A.R. and Hall, M.A. (1984). The effect of
solubilisation on the character of an ethylene-binding site from
Phaseolus vulgaris L. cotyledons. Planta 160, 474-479.

Thomas, C.J.R., Smith, A.R. and Hall, M.A. (1985). Partial purification of
an ethylene binding site from Phaseolus vulgaris L. cotyledons. Planta
164, 272-277.

Van der Linde, P.C.G., Maan, A.C., Mennes, A.M. and Libbenga, K.R. (1985). Auxin receptors in tobacco. Proc. 16th FEBS Congress, Moscow. VNU Science Press, Utrecht.

Van Rompuy, L.L.L. and Zeevaart, J.A.D. (1979). Are steroidal estrogens natural plant constituents? Phytochemistry 18, 863-865.

Veen, H. (1974). Specificity of phospholipid binding to indole acetic acid and other auxins. Z. Naturforsch. 29c, 39-41.

Veldstra, H. (1944a). Researches on plant growth substances IV. Relation between chemical structure and physiological activity I. Enzymologia 11, 97-136.

Veldstra, H. (1944b). Researches on plant growth substances IV. Relation between chemical structure and physiological activity II. Contemplations on place and mechanism of the action of the growth substances. Enzymologia 11, 137-163.

Veldstra, H. (1956). On form and function of plant growth substances. In: 'The Chemistry and Mode of Action of Plant Growth Substances'. (R.L. Wain and F. Wightman, eds.). pp 117-133. Butterworths, London.

Veluthambi, K. and Poovaiah, B.W. (1984). Polyamine-stimulated phosphorylation of proteins from corn (Zea mays L.) coleoptiles. Biochem. Biophys. Res. Commun. 122, 1374-1380.

Venis, M.A. (1971). Stimulation of RNA transcription from pea and corn DNA by protein retained on Sepharose coupled to 2,4-dichlorophenoxyacetic acid. Proc. Natl. Acad. Sci. USA 68, 1824-1827.

Venis, M.A. (1972). Auxin-induced conjugation systems in peas. Plant Physiol. 49, 24-27.

Venis, M.A. (1977a). Receptors for plant hormones. Adv. Bot. Res. 5, 53-88.

Venis, M.A. (1977b). Affinity labels for auxin binding sites in corn coleoptile membranes. Planta 134, 145-149.

Venis, M.A. (1977c). Solubilisation and partial purification of auxin-binding sites of corn membranes. Nature (London) 66, 268-269.

Venis, M.A. (1980). Purification and properties of membrane-bound auxin receptors in corn. In: 'Plant Growth Substances 1979'. (F. Skoog, ed.). pp 61-70. Springer-Verlag, Berlin - Heidelberg - New York.

Venis, M.A. (1981). Cellular recognition of plant growth regulators. In: 'Aspects and Prospects of Plant Growth Regulators'. (B. Jeffcoat, ed.). pp 187-195. Wessex Press, Wantage.

Venis, M.A. (1984). Hormone-binding studies and the misuse of precipitation assays. Planta 162, 502-505.

Van der Linde, P.C.G., Maan, A.C., Mennes, A.M. and Libbenga, K.R. (1985). Auxin receptors in tobacco. Proc. 16th FEBS Congress, Moscow. VNU Science Press, Utrecht (in press).

Van Rompuy, L.L.L. and Zeevaart, J.A.D. (1979). Are steroidal estrogens natural plant constituents? Phytochemistry 18, 863-865.

Veen, H. (1974). Specificity of phospholipid binding to indole acetic acid and other auxins. Z. Naturforsch. 29c, 39-41.

Veldstra, H. (1944a). Researches on plant growth substances IV. Relation between chemical structure and physiological activity I. Enzymologia 11, 97-136.

Veldstra, H. (1944b). Researches on plant growth substances IV. Relation between chemical structure and physiological activity II. Contemplations on place and mechanism of the action of the growth substances. Enzymologia 11, 137-163.

Veldstra, H. (1956). On form and function of plant growth substances. In: 'The Chemistry and Mode of Action of Plant Growth Substances'. (R.L. Wain and F. Wightman, eds.). pp 117-133. Butterworths, London.

Veluthambi, K. and Poovaiah, B.W. (1984). Polyamine-stimulated phosphorylation of proteins from corn (Zea mays L.) coleoptiles. Biochem. Biophys. Res. Commun. 122, 1374-1380.

Venis, M.A. (1971). Stimulation of RNA transcription from pea and corn DNA by protein retained on Sepharose coupled to 2,4-dichlorophenoxyacetic acid. Proc. Natl. Acad. Sci. USA 68, 1824-1827.

Venis, M.A. (1972). Auxin-induced conjugation systems in peas. Plant Physiol. 49, 24-27.

Venis, M.A. (1977a). Receptors for plant hormones. Adv. Bot. Res. 5, 53-88.

Venis, M.A. (1977b). Affinity labels for auxin binding sites in corn coleoptile membranes. Planta 134, 145-149.

Venis, M.A. (1977c). Solubilisation and partial purification of auxin-binding sites of corn membranes. Nature (London) 66, 268-269.

Venis, M.A. (1980). Purification and properties of membrane-bound auxin receptors in corn. In: 'Plant Growth Substnces 1979'. (F. Skoog, ed.). pp 61-70. Springer-Verlag, Berlin - Heidelberg - New York.

Venis, M.A. (1981). Cellular recognition of plant growth regulators. In: 'Aspects and Prospects of Plant Growth Regulators'. (B. Jeffcoat, ed.). pp 187-195. Wessex Press, Wantage.

Venis, M.A. (1984). Hormone-binding studies and the misuse of precipitation assays. Planta 162, 502-505.

Venis, M.A., and Watson, P.J. (1978). Naturally occurring modifiers of auxin-receptor interaction in corn: identification as benzoxazolinones. Planta 142, 103-107.

Verma, D.P.S., MacLachlan, G.A., Byrne, H. and Ewings, D. (1975). Regulation and in vitro translation of messenger ribonucleic acid for cellulase from auxin-treated pea epicotyls. J. Biol. Chem. 250, 1019-1026.

Vreugdenhil, D., Burgers, A. and Libbenga, K.R. (1979). A particle-bound auxin receptor from tobacco pith callus. Plant Sci. Lett. 16, 115-121.

Vreugdenhil, D., Harkes, P.A.A. and Libbenga, K.R. (1980). Auxin-binding by particulate fractions from tobacco leaf protoplasts. Planta 150, 9-12.

Vreugdenhil, D., Burgers, A., Harkes, P.A.A. and Libbenga, K.R. (1981). Modulation of the number of membrane-bound auxin-binding sites during the growth of batch-cultured tobacco cells. Planta 152, 415-419.

Wada, K., Marumo, S., Ikekawa, N., Morisaki, M. and Mori, K. (1981). Brassinolide and homobrassinolide promotion of lamina inclination of rice seedlings. Plant Cell Physiol. 22, 323-325.

Walker, J.C. and Key, J.L. (1982). Isolation of cloned cDNAs to auxin-responsive poly(A)[+]RNAs of elongating soybean hypocotyl. Proc. Natl. Acad. Sci. USA 79, 7185-7189.

Walton, J.D. and Ray, P.M. (1981). Evidence for receptor function of auxin binding sites in maize. Plant Physiol. 68, 1334-1338.

Wardrop, A.J. and Polya, G.M. (1977). Properties of a soluble auxin-binding protein from dwarf bean seedlings. Plant Sci. Lett. 8, 155-163.

Wardrop, A.J. and Polya, G.M. (1980). Co-purification of pea and bean leaf soluble auxin-binding protein with ribulose-1,5-bisphosphate carboxylase. Plant Physiol. 66, 105-111.

Weigl, J. (1969). Einbau von Auxin in gequollene Lecithin-Lamellen. Z. Naturforsch. 24B, 365-366.

Welshons, W.V., Liebermann, M.E. and Gorski, J. (1984). Nuclear localization of unoccupied oestrogen receptors. Nature (London) 307, 747-749.

Wilchek, M., Salomon, Y., Lowe, M. and Selinger, Z. (1971). Conversion of protein kinase to a cyclic AMP independent form by affinity chromatography on N[6]-caproyl 3',5'-cyclic adenosine monophosphate-Sepharose. Biochem. Biophys. Res. Commun. 45, 1177-1184.

Wilchek, M., Miron, T. and Kohn, J. (1984). Affinity chromatography. Methods in Enzymology 104, 3-55.

Williamson, F.A., Morré, D.J. and Hess, K. (1977). Auxin binding activities of subcellular fractions from soybean hypocotyls. Cytobiologie 16, 63-71.

Wong, J.R. and Sussex, I.M. (1980). Isolation of abscisic acid resistant variants from tobacco cell cultures II. Selection and characterization of variants. Planta 148, 103-107.

Wood, A. and Paleg, L.G. (1972). The influence of gibberellic acid on the permeability of model membrane systems. Plant Physiol. 50, 103-108.

Wood, A. and Paleg, L.G. (1974). Alteration of liposomal membrane fluidity by gibberellic acid. Aust. J. Plant Physiol. 1, 31-40.

Yokota, T., Arima, M. and Takahashi, N. (1982a). Castasterone, a new phytosterol with plant-hormone potency, from chestnut insect gall. Tetrahedron Lett. 23, 1275-1278.

Yokota, T., Baba, J. and Takahashi, N. (1982b). A new steroidal lactone with plant growth-regulatory activity from Dolichos lablab seed. Tetrahedron Lett. 23, 4965-4966.

Yokota, T., Morita, M. and Takahashi, N. (1983). 6-Deoxocastasterone and 6-deoxodolichosterone: putative precursors for brassinolide-related steroids from Phaseolus vulgaris. Agric. Biol. Chem. 47, 2149-2151.

Yoshida, K. and Takegami,T. (1977). Isolation of cytokinin-binding protein from tobacco leaves by bioaffinity chromatography and its partial characterization. J. Biochem. (Tokyo) 81, 791-799.

Yu, Y.-B., Adams, D.O. and Yang, S.F. (1979). Regulation of auxin-induced ethylene production in mung bean hypocotyls. Plant Physiol. 63, 589-590.

Zazimalova, E. and Kutacek, M. (1985a). In vitro binding of auxin to particulate fractions from the shoots of dark-grown wheat seedlings. Plant Growth Regul. 3, 15-26.

Zazimalova, E. and Kutacek, M. (1985b). Auxin-binding site in wheat shoots: interactions between indol-3ylacetic acid and its halogenated derivatives. Biologia Plant. (in press).

Zocchi, G., Rogers, S.A. and Hanson, J.B. (1983). Inhibition of proton pumping in corn roots is associated with increased phosphorylation of membrane proteins. Plant Sci. Lett. 31, 215-221.

Zurfluh, L.L. and Guilfoyle, T.J. (1982a). Auxin-induced changes in the population of translatable messenger RNA in elongating sections of soybean hypocotyl. Plant Physiol. 69, 332-337.

Zurfluh, L.L. and Guilfoyle, T.J. (1982b). Auxin- and ethylene-induced changes in the population of translatable messenger RNA in basal sections and intact soybean hypocotyl. Plant Physiol. 69, 338-340.

Index